1 Psychological ideas in speech and language therapy

Introduction

Speech and language therapy draws enormously from other disciplines including linguistics and phonetics, medical sciences and, perhaps most of all, psychology. Whilst few may disagree with the idea that both academic and applied elements of psychology play important roles in the practice of speech and language therapy, there may be a variety of views about how much psychology, in what form and whether it has been sufficiently examined in relation to the needs of adults and children with communication and swallowing difficulties.

Developmental and cognitive psychology have a critical role to play in speech and language therapy practice, enabling us to understand how to identify typical and atypical human development and the ways in which cognitive processes such as memory and executive function impact upon language and communication. Over the past 25 years or so, the fields of psycholinguistics and cognitive neuropsychology have illuminated the processes by which speech and language is produced and understood, and these developments have enabled the profession to make significant advances in diagnosing the precise nature of speech and language breakdown and are beginning to offer new treatment possibilities.

The focus of this book is on different areas of psychology to those outlined above. Speech and language therapy practice might be viewed in terms of a triad (Figure 1.1). All students and practitioners learn and use technical knowledge and skills related to speech, language and swallowing problems. They can apply theory to hypothesize about the nature of their clients' communication and swallowing difficulties. They know how to conduct and interpret assessments and how to use their findings to select and evaluate appropriate interventions. These are important and unique aspects of the speech and language therapist's role. Nevertheless, despite this highly-skilled activity, many speech and language therapists observe that different clients vary enormously in their response to the same intervention. On the part of the client, avoidance, lack of awareness, understanding or motivation, inability or unwillingness to change, high levels of anxiety or feelings of loss and grief may all influence therapeutic outcome.

At the same time, the effect of the therapist him- or herself on speech and language therapy outcomes also needs careful consideration; no doubt many readers will be able to reflect upon their experiences of professionals they have encountered over the course of their lives – teachers, lecturers, doctors and so on – and how their feelings about the particular *individual* have influenced their willingness to engage with and act upon their guidance. This book concerns itself both with what Fourie (2009) describes as "therapeutic qualities and actions which support the therapeutic relationship", and with "technical knowledge and skills that facilitate change and coping for our clients" (Figure 1.1). These areas of practice draw particularly on an understanding and application of ideas from health and counselling psychology, drawing on medical and psychotherapeutic literature. It also considers some areas of social psychology, an understanding of which provides an important insight into how we can best work with clients holistically.

In her book, *Scientific Thinking in Speech and Language Therapy*, Carmel Lum (2001) reflects on science and art in intervention. Characteristics associated with science include 'micro', evidence base, content, prescriber, rule governed,

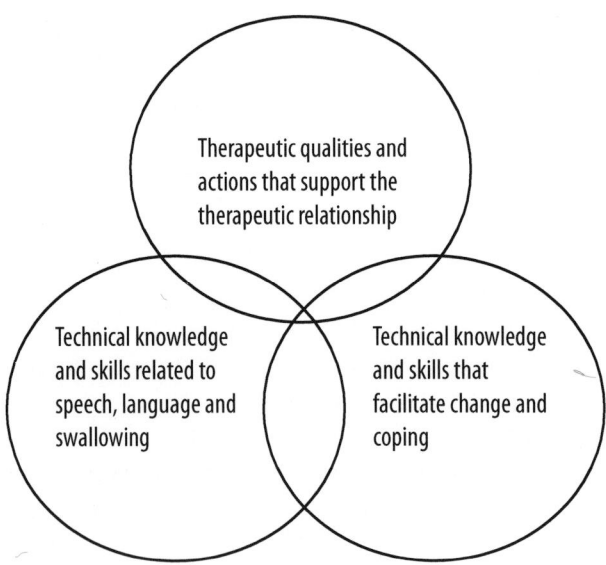

Figure 1.1 The scope of speech and language therapy practice.

Applying
Psychological Ideas
in
Speech and Language Therapy

British Library Cataloguing in Publication Data

A catalogue record for this book is available from the British Library

Cover design: Jim Wilkie

Cover image used under license from Shutterstock.com

Project management, typesetting and design: J&R Publishing Services Ltd, Guildford, Surrey, UK; www.jr-publishingservices.co.uk

Printed and bound by CPI Group (UK) Ltd, Croydon, CR0 4YY

Applying Psychological Ideas in Speech and Language Therapy

Sarah James and Shelagh Brumfitt

J&R Press Ltd

Contents

data collection, hypothesis testing, evaluating, replicable, doable by anyone with 'the instructions'. The qualities of the scientist – perhaps analogous to the 'pathologist' – include rigour, intellect, logic. The art (or *therapy*) of practice is more likely to embody words such as holistic, intuition, therapeutic alliance, healer, creativity, the talents of specific individuals, and 'the x-factor'.

Over recent years, there has been a great emphasis on the scientific aspects of speech and language therapy. The profession has embraced – and rightly so – evidence-based practice; it is necessary for our survival. Lum is ultimately making the case for applying scientific reasoning in speech and language therapy practice. Nonetheless, she does not see the art and science of practice as mutually exclusive and writes eloquently on the 'art' of speech and language therapy:

> "…therapy is still based on an interaction between at least two or more people. Therapy is an interaction between people that involves a gesture of healing as well as the difficult-to-define qualities of trust, hope, faith, charisma, affect, empathy and kindness. A therapeutic relationship between the clinician and the patient possesses an ethereal quality and is inaccessible to others."
>
> *Lum, 2001, p.225*

Whilst understanding the thought behind Lum's characterization of the therapeutic relationship as 'ethereal' and 'inaccessible', we would also argue that there is much that can be said and learned about it. The dichotomy between science and art is, in many ways, a false one and scientific understanding,

---

Box 1.1 Science and art

In the UK, the name of professionals who work with people who have speech, language or swallowing difficulties is speech and language therapist. In some other English-speaking countries, notably the US and Australia, they are referred to as speech or speech-language pathologist. Reflecting on these titles, do they seem to have different connotations? Is there a tension between them or might both elements always be present, with the balance between them shifting in different circumstances, with different clients, clinicians, and therapeutic approaches or at different stages in the therapeutic process? Do you prefer one over another? Why? Where do you naturally see yourself on the spectrum of artist and scientist?

particularly of psychological theory, can illuminate many aspects of therapy practice.

Psychology in education, practice and research

To qualify as a speech and language therapist, it is necessary to develop knowledge and understanding about a wide range of topics, possibly more wide ranging in content than in other professions. Alongside and underpinning being an expert in human communication disorders, a speech and language therapist must be a biomedical scientist, a linguist, a phonetician and a psychologist, amongst others. These foundations of the professional subject have built up over many years to inform and create specific interventions covering the scope of practice, so that a knowledge of the anatomical structure, the linguistic features and the psychological attitude of an individual all contribute to therapeutic decisions. These subject requirements are reflected in the professional regulations used to approve speech and language therapy education and practice. Current Health and Care Professions Council (HCPC) Standards of Proficiency (http://www. hpc-uk.org/assets/documents/10000529Standards_of_Proficiency_SLTs. pdf) refer to required knowledge across the disciplines of linguistics and phonetics, the understanding of biomedical and medical sciences in relation to communication and swallowing, the understanding of psychology as relevant to lifespan development, psychological and social wellbeing and an understanding of sociology including its application to educational, health and workplace settings (HCPC, Standards of Proficiency, 2014). The Royal College of Speech and Language Therapists in its Curriculum Guidelines (2018) has similar requirements. Internationally, these requirements are recognized in the profession of speech and language therapy in New Zealand (https:// speechtherapy.org.nz/about-slt/), speech and language pathology in Australia (https://www.speechpathologyaustralia.org.au/), the USA (http://www.asha. org/) and Canada (http://www.sac-oac.ca) and orthophonie and logopaedics across mainland Europe (http://www.cplol.eu/profession/general-info.html). All accredited university courses are required to teach the 'basic disciplines', along with the complete range of communication difficulties, their assessment and approaches to intervention. As teaching and assessment methods have evolved, what has been noticeable over time is the way the educational reading material has developed for students; there are now many textbooks focused on specific communication and swallowing difficulties. Biomedical sciences have produced relevant textbooks for students. Linguistics and phonetics are represented in impressive quantities of texts with direct application to speech and language therapy, developments which also reflect increased research in the area.

It is our observation that the textbooks which cover the range of required material in the field of psychology have emerged in a rather different way. Where linguistics and phonetics have provided a clear route from theory to the practice of speech and language therapy, the link from psychology has been less clear and the literature more limited. Specific topics have been dealt with, such as the role of cognitive psychology in the understanding of aphasia or how the framework for child development informs our understanding of developmental speech and language disorder. However, knowledge of social and health psychology has not been so frequently or explicitly applied to speech and language therapy and direct discussion of how this fits into practice is generally only found in specific writings or clinical guidance. This may well reflect the evolving nature both of the profession and of health care more widely. For example, speech and language therapists may increasingly find themselves working in a context where direct 'face to face' time with clients, involving detailed analysis of speech and language, is limited by service frameworks and where the role of clients themselves as 'self-managers' is emphasized. In these circumstances, it is imperative that strategies for maximizing the effectiveness of this relatively new way of practising are identified and applied.

There has been a considerable amount of research around the psychosocial impact of communication and (to a much lesser extent) swallowing difficulties. Such research, often qualitative in nature, adds significantly to our understanding of what it means for a person to have a communication difficulty and the potential impact that it has on their wellbeing, relationships and occupational lives. It forms an important strand of the evidence base and points to the importance of foregrounding the whole person over the communication or swallowing impairment. Less well understood is *what* might be done and *how* and whether doing one thing is any more *effective* than doing another – or nothing at all – in terms of improving therapy outcomes. Time and again, literature searches for key concepts discussed in this book (for example, 'adherence'; 'therapeutic alliance') yield, at most, a bare handful of results when combined with 'speech and language therapy' and its variants. Even the few papers that do directly address the role of psychology in speech and language therapy tend to be confined to relatively few contexts, probably the most notable of these being stammering or voice disorders. It is therefore important to acknowledge that empirical research into the application of the psychological ideas discussed here in wider speech and language therapy practice is limited, a state of affairs that we hope will change over the coming years.

The aims of this book

Meleis (2011) discusses the idea of 'borrowed theory', stating that *"knowledge does not innately 'belong' to any field of science"* (Meleis, p.131). However, she also argues that theories from other disciplines must be adapted to the professional 'milieu' in order to be meaningful to that profession. Discussing nursing, she writes:

> "Even when theories developed in other disciplines are used to explain nursing phenomena, and nursing problems, the new derivations and new syntheses make them nursing theories. …Nursing theories evolve out of the practice arena or anything that pertains to the practice arena. They are then tested in research. Until the time-consuming job of research is accomplished, the face validity of a theory, as it pertains to practice, should be enough to be a blueprint for action."
>
> *Meleis, 2011, p.131*

Psychological ideas are amongst the many borrowed theories in the discipline of speech and language therapy. Owing to our own careers in universities and our experience in teaching both clinical and theoretical material to students, we have been aware for some time that there needed to be a broader selection of psychological material for professionals and students alike to use in guiding clinical practice. The book is not intended – nor could it be – a comprehensive guide to health, social or counselling psychology. Rather, we have sought to summarize and signpost a set of relevant psychological perspectives, highlighting examples of literature where these have been applied in related contexts such as medicine and nursing, counselling and allied health professions, and providing suggestions for practical application in speech and language therapy. In doing so, we hope to draw attention to theories that can address the '*what*' and '*how*' aspects of applying psychological ideas in practice, that have face validity and that have potential to provide a 'blueprint' for action, pending research to investigate them.

The chapters: Aims and content

Each chapter within this book explores a different aspect of social, health and counselling psychology. Chapter 2, Being Therapeutic, addresses the components, features and behaviours found in the act of therapy. The concept of being person-centred is explored using a framework (Mead & Bower, 2000) which, though developed as a way of understanding the doctor–patient relationship, offers a structure and ideas that resonate strongly with speech and language therapy practice. The unique characteristics of the client and the professional are considered along with the interaction between them; the therapeutic alliance drawing on literature from medicine, psychotherapy and allied health professional as well as our own. Leading on from this, the common factors model and its application to speech and language therapy is discussed. Also considered in this chapter are some practical factors that might influence person-centeredness and the therapeutic relationship, focusing particularly on cultural contexts and the role of technology in contemporary practice. Finally, the process of discharge is explored in terms of its impact on both the client and therapist.

Chapter 3 considers personal and social change across the lifespan, providing an overview of a range of psychosocial explanations for lifespan development using the works of Erikson (1968), Bronfenbrenner (1979) and Hendry and Kloep (2002). Each of these takes a different but complementary approach to understanding human development by providing insight into how individuals move through the ageing process, the contextual factors that are influential in this process and the way in which challenges faced along the way can lead to personal growth or decay. This chapter includes material on different phases of the lifespan, looking at the challenge of disability in the context of different age groups and considers how disability can both influence and be influenced by the ageing process.

In Chapter 4, the focus is on the technical skills and knowledge which facilitate adherence and behaviour change and argues that an understanding of these is core to successful therapy outcomes in the context of modern healthcare practice with its focus on client responsibility and self-management. The chapter outlines a number of models and ideas, drawn from counselling, health psychology and coaching literature, that have been used to understand and promote behaviour change and shows how they have been, or could be, applied in a speech and language therapy context.

The theme of 'client characteristics', introduced in Chapter 2, is considered from a different perspective at the start of Chapter 5 by exploring the concept of illness perceptions. The potential importance of the *therapist* understanding how the *client* understands his or her difficulties (or those of a child or other family member) is discussed alongside suggestions for ways in which this can be achieved. The chapter then turns to a discussion of stress and coping, considered from the perspective of both client and the therapist. In the final part of the chapter, some ideas and applications from the field of positive psychology are introduced. These are drawn from the work of Martin Seligman and colleagues as well as from broader concepts such as resilience, optimism and hope, echoing some of the themes that were introduced in Chapter 2.

Finally, Chapter 6 focuses more closely on the practical components of therapy, particularly in the context of wellbeing, and how this may be managed. The role of counselling in speech and language therapy is discussed along with guidance on some of the skills and methods required. Extending out from the basic skills, the chapter moves to cover some explicit methods, such as Solution Focused Brief Therapy, Cognitive Behaviour Therapy and Narrative Therapy.

Within each chapter, there are boxes which contain brief clinical vignettes, invitations to reflect on professional qualities and practice as well as practical exercises that serve to illustrate the application of the ideas and theories presented within the text. In some instances, we have added our own ideas to these whilst in others, mindful of the broad range of practice, we have intentionally omitted these so that the reader is free to apply ideas in his or her own particular context.

Common themes and tensions

The themes of 'therapeutic relationships and qualities' and 'skills that facilitate change' are interwoven throughout the chapters. They are, in many ways, inseparable; the therapeutic relationship is itself an important agent for change and, at the same time, strategies to support clients in the process of change are probably more likely to be successful in the context of a strong therapeutic relationship. Nevertheless, as are highlighted in Chapters 2 and 4, there may be occasions when there is potential for tension between the two. Whilst therapeutic change is desirable, it is important not to assume that this concept is identical to 'behaviour change', 'self-management' or even 'client-empowerment'. If the speech and language therapist, however skilfully, continuously pushes an agenda of clients 'doing things for themselves' and fails to recognize when the client does not want this or is not ready for it, the therapeutic relationship is likely to suffer. Perhaps, then, an understanding of when to focus on change and when simply to listen is one of the most important skills at the heart of therapy practice.

These ideas are thoughtfully discussed by Owens (2015) who differentiates two notions of 'personal' in the healthcare system. On the one hand, patients and clients are involved in the planning, delivery and evaluation of their own care (through, for example, shared decision making, personal healthcare budgets and patient outcome measures such as the family and friends test). Beyond this, he argues, the notion of patient empowerment is closely associated with that of 'self-management' particularly for people with chronic conditions (e.g., Collins & Rochfort, 2016). Thus, 'personalization' changes the NHS *"from a service that does thing to or for its patients to one which does things either with patients or provides them with an opportunity to do things for themselves"* (Owens, 2015, p.25).

The other type of personalization described by Owens is the intimate relationship between professional and patient which involves trust, understanding and empathy and attending to the emotional and psychological aspects of the patient as well as the physical, an idea that seems to be closely aligned with 'therapeutic alliance'. Owens (2015, pp.26–28) discusses a number of ways in which these two ideas about personalization may be in conflict with each other. For example:

- The introduction of market forces may 'crowd out' existing social norms and values that were previously prevalent (Sandel, 2009, cited in Owens, 2015). For example, the notions of choice, independence and convenience associated with the first definition of personalization may result in a transactional set of norms and an element of commodification in the patient–professional relationship. Patients may be seen as a source of revenue to professionals and a trip to the GP – or speech and language therapist – may be seen in a similar light as a trip to the shops. The roles of both professionals and clients may be 'recast', with the patient as 'a consumer, customer, service user' and the professional as 'care plan manager, information provider, gatekeeper to resources' (Owens, 2015, p.28).

- The emphasis on demand and supply and outputs (number of contacts, discharges, etc.), administrative protocols (Cribb, 2011, cited in Owens, 2015) and tightly-controlled care pathways may have the effect of eroding the agency (not to mention the time) needed to develop an empathetic and intimate patient–professional relationship.

Mol (2008, cited in Owens, 2015, p28) compares the principles governing markets, breaking up components and assigning a value so that cost comparisons can be made with those of healthcare which he sees as open ended and uncertain, not fitting well with the quantifiable metrics of the market. Whereas 'good practice' is framed in the language of choice and autonomy, there may be other models of professional practice (and, arguably perhaps, this includes speech and language therapy) where there is limited choice but high-quality care is delivered through close professional relationships. There is an assumed primacy in the value of choice but this may be at the expense of trust and intimacy (Owens, 2015, p.29). Furthermore, for choice to be meaningful, there must be realistic options that can be acted upon. This may not always be the case, for example, where someone has a chronic or degenerative illness, where there is not more than one 'evidence-based' option, or where limited resources are rationed in order to deliver services equitably. For example, in speech and language therapy, it is unlikely that a parent would be given a meaningful choice between bringing their child to a language group or having individual 1:1 therapy. These arguments – as much in the realm of the political and economic as the psychological – are worth reflecting on because they highlight a possible tension between two key aspects that run as themes through this book, namely sharing power and responsibility and the therapeutic alliance. Both these ideas 'feel' valuable. Yet many speech and language therapists may recognize how elements from Owens' discussion, such as structured pathways, limited resources and the 'business' of healthcare have the potential to influence the way we construe our professional identity, our roles and the personal relationships that we have with clients.

Who is the book for?

Its first role is to provide an additional source for students in speech and language therapy whether at the pre-registration or post-graduate level including PhD students. However, we also hope that this material provides useful perspectives which the experienced therapist can draw upon. It may form the basis for a debate about the role of social and health psychology because, for us as authors, surprised that this material is not more overtly part of practice.

The psychology material in this book can be found in a wide range of psychology, sociology and psychology textbooks. However, the linking together of this material with its application to speech and language therapy is much rarer. The book therefore brings together sources of information which may be used by current and future therapists to enhance practice. We believe that the changing nature of speech and language therapy practice makes the application of psychological ideas within it more relevant now than ever. We hope that this book will increase awareness and insight of how this can happen and prompt further discussion, debate and publication in this area.

Note on terminology

Before continuing, it will be useful to say a few words about terminology. Literature focusing on the medical profession tends to use the terms 'physician' or 'doctor' and 'patient'. In a broader context, the term 'health professional' or 'professional' is often used. Some (mainly medical) literature refers to 'patient-centred care', though our preferred term is 'person-centred care'. Within the speech and language 'profession' itself, the terms 'pathologist' (SLP) or 'therapist' (SLT) are used, depending on the source being discussed. Within this book, when discussing specific literature, we use the terms used within that literature but invite readers to look beyond these. Our own preferred terms are 'therapist' or 'SLT' and 'client'.

2 Being therapeutic

Introduction

As speech and language therapists, we work with an enormous variety of clients in many different settings. Sometimes our relationships with them may be very brief; we may see them once when doing a hospital bedside swallow assessment or a community clinic triage. Alternatively, the relationship may extend over many months or even years, such as when working with children with complex needs and their families, or with people who have degenerative illnesses. Working with people is at the heart of what we do; indeed, wanting to work with people is usually one of the first things that applicants to pre-registration speech and language therapy courses will say has attracted them to the profession. We are neither doctors nor counsellors, yet both of these professions have something in common with our own and the way we conceptualize our practice in relation to them can inform the way we interact and form relationships with our clients. This interaction, in turn, has the potential to be a powerful influence – perhaps *the* most powerful influence – on therapeutic outcomes.

The relationship between healthcare professionals and patients or clients has been explored from many different perspectives. Some ideas focus on the *role* of the health professional – and, indeed, clients - within the context of the relationship whilst others propose models or frameworks which seek to explain the processes by which relationships are formed and factors which impact upon these processes. Not surprisingly, given its long history, the nature of relationships between clients and health professionals has been explored extensively through the lens of the medical profession and the 'physician–patient' relationship. In modern times, the emergence of psychology and its application to this relationship has been highly influential in developing the way it is understood and in bringing to the fore the power of the professional *themselves* (as opposed to the drug or other intervention) in bringing about change in patients. In the 1960s, Balint, a doctor and psychotherapist, maintained that "the most powerful tool the doctor possessed was himself or herself" (Kaba & Sooriakumaran, 2007, p.60), an idea that has been discussed extensively in the psychotherapy and counselling literature in the context of the 'therapeutic relationship'. At the same time, in Western cultures at least, the role of the patient has shifted from passive recipient of healthcare in a paternalistic model in which the healthcare professional acts as 'guardian' (Emanuel & Emanuel, 1992) to that of 'partner' or, latterly, 'service-user', in an era of personalization, choice and person-centred care. These two overlapping ideas – the power of the relationship and patient- or person-centred care – form the focus of this chapter, which reflects upon how ideas from medicine and counselling, from other health professions and our own, can illuminate the relationship between speech and language therapists and their clients.

Being person-centred

Aside from political and moral rationales there are a number of reasons for providing person-centred care. DiLollo and Favreau (2010) discuss patient-centred care in the context of evidence-based speech and language therapy practice as being closely associated with patient values. In an era of 'client as consumer' (epitomized in the NHS by innovations such as the 'family and friends test') it has been shown that those receiving patient-centred care tend to be more satisfied, to perceive the quality of care they receive as being higher and to have outcomes (Mead & Bower, 2002). Finally, the concept of patient-centred care, particularly Mead and Bower's dimensions of 'therapeutic alliance' and 'doctor as person', described below, is intertwined with the notion of 'common factors'. This is discussed in more detail later in the chapter but, in essence, refers to the idea, discussed extensively within the psychotherapeutic literature, that clinician effects are at least as powerful – and perhaps more so – than treatment effects (e.g., Wampold, 2015).

DiLollo and Favreau discuss the question of whether speech and language pathologists *do* indeed provide patient-centred care. They are writing from a US perspective and the very title of the profession – 'pathologist' – together with the language of intervention, such as 'diagnosis' and 'treatment plan' hints at a dominant medical model (DiLollo & Favreau, 2010). Interventions are often highly structured or manualized and tend to emphasize the role of clinician as 'teacher' and client as 'error maker'. Later in the chapter, we look a little more closely at the discourse of therapy and its implications for the therapist–client relationship.

In one of the only explicit empirical investigations of person-centred care in speech and language therapy, DiLollo and Favreau (2010) report a pilot study comparing the person-centred behaviours of first and second year graduate speech and language pathology clinicians in the US. Although findings were inconclusive, the authors identified the interesting point that students perceived that their clinic grade was more heavily influenced by their technical skills than by their person-centeredness, a consequence of the grading form which was developed from the ASHA Standards. Similarly, in the UK, the HCPC Standards of Proficiency inform the clinical grading criteria for many pre-registration courses; the large proportion of the standards relate to discipline or technical knowledge or to professional requirements such as record keeping. DiLollo and Favreau refer to Geller & Foley (2009) who suggest that supervision practices in speech and language therapy *"tend to focus on concrete, discipline-specific knowledge and skills at the expense of 'other kinds of knowledge' such as psychodynamic, intrapersonal, subjective and affective"* (DiLollo & Favreau, 2010, p.23). These findings resonate with those of a somewhat similar study undertaken with occupational therapy students. Bonsaksen (2013) used The Intentional Relationship Model (IRM) (Taylor, 2008) to explore occupational therapy (OT) students' preferences for ways of relating to clients and is discussed a little later in the chapter. The 'problem-solving' mode was the most preferred and Bonsaken hypothesizes that this may be because novice OTs tend to operate more comfortably within a medical model, seeing the client as having a defined 'problem' which the therapists can help to 'fix'. This analysis certainly resonates with our own experiences of working with speech and language therapy students. For example, when participating in simulated client sessions (in which actors play the part of clients or carers), students are guided to use skills which support the development of a therapeutic relationship and view clients and carers as experts, able to develop their own solutions. Nevertheless, students' drive to offer suggestions, solve problems and provide a 'right answer' is often overwhelming at this stage in their development as speech and language therapists.

The meaning of person-centred care

Although there is fairly limited explicit literature on person-centred care within speech and language therapy, examining practice through the lens of a conceptual framework can provide a useful means of exploring and understanding practice. Mead & Bower (2000) developed an empirically-based framework of patient-centred care and the factors that influence it. Although focused upon the *doctor*-patient relationship in its original conception, the framework has been considered 'seminal' and been widely cited within the healthcare literature (Kitson, Marshall, Bassett, & Zeitz, 2013). Mead and

Bower themselves note that the applicability of their model to disciplines other than medicine warrants further exploration. Nevertheless, with this caveat in mind, this chapter uses the model as an organizing framework for considering the relationships that we have with clients. Mead and Bower's framework is by no means the only model of patient-centeredness but it is undoubtedly one of the most comprehensive. It contains many useful and familiar ideas for reflecting upon the meaning of being person-centred within our own profession and many related ideas, for example models of professional client relationships; shared decision making and common factors can easily be considered within the dimensions of the framework. It also provides a coherent means of navigating through the many different approaches and varying use of terms that have been taken to exploring the relationship between health professionals and their clients. So, although speech and language therapy does not itself have an extensive literature that specifically or empirically considers 'the therapist–client relationship' or 'person-centred care', the framework can help to signpost studies and ideas that are nonetheless relevant.

Five dimensions of patient-centred care are identified within the framework: the biopsychosocial model; the 'patient as person'; sharing power and responsibility; the therapeutic alliance; and 'doctor as person'. Under each broad heading, the concepts originally described in Mead and Bowers' framework are described below and extended to discuss ideas from the wider literature in the context of speech and language therapy practice.

The biopsychosocial perspective

The biopsychosocial perspective provides a context for patient-centred care by extending the health professional's arena of interest beyond the biological to include the psychological and social domains. The patient-centred health professional has a "willingness to become involved in the full range of difficulties patients bring ... and not just their biomedical problems" (Stewart et al., 1995, cited in Mead & Bowers, 2000). The importance of being open to the client's 'hidden agenda' (Lipkin et al., 1984, cited in Kaba & Sooriakumaran, 2007) is recognized. Speech and language therapists are likely to be highly familiar with principles associated with the biopsychosocial model. In most settings, working with a client holistically underpins their work; speech and language therapists usually strive to understand the impact of communication and swallowing difficulties on the person and the social systems within which they operate and work and with clients and their families towards functional outcomes (not simply the 'impairment'). The idea of 'quality of life' is closely associated with the biopsychosocial model. At the time of writing, an ad hoc literature search (Medline; CINHAL and PsychInfo) using the search terms 'speech and language therapy' and 'quality of life' revealed in excess of 1450 papers. The biopsychosocial model is epitomized by the International Classification of Functioning, Disability and Health (ICF) of the World Health Organisation, a framework for measuring health and disability. It considers impairment (for example, dysarthria), activity limitations (for example, holding a conversation in a noisy environment), participation restriction (for example, socialising with friends in the pub) and wellbeing (for example, feeling lonely). Enderby's *Therapy Outcome Measures* (TOMs), widely used in speech and language therapy as well as other health professions, are based on the ICF (Enderby & John, 2015).

In addition to reflecting a holistic view of working with clients, the biopsychosocial model is also closely associated with the idea that the health professional works with 'healthy' people, potentially at a population level through, for example, health promotion. The work of speech and language therapists working in Sure Start Programmes, prevalent in the 1990 and 2000s providing services targeting at-risk groups, contains many examples of health promotion (Fuller, 2010). Law, Reilly, and Snow (2013) argue that speech and language therapy services need to be grounded in public health principles in order to provide appropriate prevention and intervention services to meet the need of the population. Ferguson and Spence (2012) interviewed speech and language therapists to explore what 'health promotion' meant to them. Participants particularly focused on their role of 'education and enablement' of others to assume responsibility for speech, language and communication development and saw this as a way of maximizing limited resources. Providing education was seen as a key way of achieving this, particularly through training of, for example, healthcare workers, education workers, carers or parents. One of the participants highlights the implication of this increasingly important speech and language therapy role for the education of speech and language therapy students and many courses include training skills as part of their curricula (Ferguson & Spence, 2012, p.529) to meet modern workforce needs.

Sharing power and responsibility

This dimension encapsulates the move away from the paternalistic model and characterizes the patient as an 'active consumer' of health care with rights such as access to information and being actively involved in treatment decisions. Shared decision making is an important way in which power and responsibility can be shared in the professional–client relationship. It is a key part of NHS strategy for improving patient experience ('No decision about me without me') and numerous resources for patients, professionals and commissioners can be found online (https://www.england.nhs.uk/ourwork/pe/sdm/). The NHS Choice Framework (https://www.gov.uk/government/publications/the-nhs-choice-framework/the-nhs-choice-framework-what-choices-are-available-to-me-in-the-nhs) identifies nine choices that are available to patients, including choosing to have a personal health budget and choosing services provided in the community. Aside from the ideological principles behind this notion, there is also some evidence to associate it with improved patient outcomes, particularly understanding, satisfaction and trust (Shay & Lafata, 2015).

Shared decision making is usually described as involving a number of steps. In her discussion of shared decision making in the medical aspects of stroke, Armstrong (2017, p.2) summarizes these as:

Step 1: Engaging the client (and other decision makers, such as family or other professionals) in the decision-making process.

Step 2: Clearly describing the options available, including potential benefits and risks, as well uncertainty.

Step 3: Assessing the client's values and goals in relation to the various options. These might reflect cultural values (these are discussed further later in the chapter) as well as priorities, such as quality of life, efficacy and so on.

Step 4: Making the decision together.

There has been little exploration of the role of shared decision making in speech and language therapy, although in 2014 it was the focus of a keynote speech by Hilary Bekker at the RCSLT conference. Bekker noted that, in general, shared decision making frequently happens in a rather limited way; professionals give information about a procedure or therapy and patients give their values and ask questions based on the professional's cue. Although professionals produce more and more information, patients report not having a choice and not being informed (Legare, 2014, cited by Bekker, 2014). She reports work on decision aids that help people to make informed choices between options which encourage people to use 'system 2' decision making (Kahneman, 2011). This deliberative-analytic and slow form of decision making involves attending to the details of the problem, evaluating the pros and cons of all options and making a choice based on 'trade-offs' between evaluations. Although it is time-consuming and more emotionally demanding, it results in more stable values and choices and fewer regrets (Bekker, 2014). Bekker argues that patients *and* staff use system 1 (intuitive, fast and using a 'rule of thumb' approach that is influenced by experiences and beliefs). Many examples of decision aids for a variety of health conditions, including multiple sclerosis, glue ear and stroke prevention, are available online. Bekker notes the challenges for implementing shared decision making in speech and language therapy; the evidence base for therapy options for many conditions is unclear, the evidence of the benefits and burdens (acceptability) of different therapy options from clients' perspectives is unclear and the use of written and other information-based support for clients with communication difficulties may be challenging. Whilst it is undoubtedly true that structured and 'information-heavy' approaches to shared decision making may be inappropriate for some clients, speech and language therapists are also skilled in using strategies such as Total Communication as well as structured approaches such as Talking Mats, developed by Joan Murphy (http://www.talkingmats.com/) when working with clients to elicit preferences and feedback.

Aside from the questions of how shared decision making can be facilitated, it is also important to consider whether this is something that is invariably seen as desirable by clients. Watts Pappas, McAllister, and McLeod, (2016) explored the beliefs and experiences of parents about their involvement in intervention for children with speech sound disorder in the context of a family-centred practice approach. They discuss previous work which tended to show that parents see the professional as the primary decision maker and provider of intervention and were ambivalent about their own level of involvement (Carroll, 2010, cited in Watts Pappas et al., 2016). In some cases, misunderstandings about the type and level of involvement expected had led to dissatisfaction (Glogowska & Campbell, 2000, cited in Watts Pappas et al., 2016). As with previous studies, Watts Pappas and colleagues found that, although parents overwhelmingly wanted to 'do right' by their child they did not expect, prior to attending therapy, to be 'overly involved' and tended to prefer the SLT to take the lead as illustrated by this quote, taken from the study:

> Doug: To me it's just like going to the quack [doctor] you know. You go along and you say you know 'the kid's got these symptoms' and you let the quack deal with it. You go

home and do these exercises, take this or do that. As for being partners, I don't know about that.

Interviewer: And would you like it to be a partnership?

Doug: Well, I don't see how it can be a partnership when you're dealing with professional people. It's their job, you can't tell them what to do. You can't take your car to the mechanic and be a partner with the mechanic, can you?

Watts Pappas et al., 2016, pp.235–236

Overall, the data from this small sample suggested that "*As long as the parents trusted and liked their SLTs they were satisfied to allow them to go about 'fixing' their child*" (Watts Pappas et al., 2016, p.236). The authors hypothesize that, to some extent, this view may reflect the 'non-pervasive' nature of the communication difficulty (mild to moderate speech sound disorder). They recommend that prior discussion about the roles of professionals and parents, matching activities to goals and discussing the benefits of parent involvement, is likely to support understanding of what is expected and willingness to be more involved. They also refer to the important question of whether SLTs should insist on family involvement in decision making and suggest that a family/person-centred approach ultimately means accepting the choice of the family about their level of involvement, whilst also being aware that willingness to be involved may increase over time as they become more familiar with the service (Forsingdal et al., 2013, cited in Watts Pappas et al., 2016).

The 'patient-as-person'

The 'patient as person' dimension is related to the biopsychosocial perspective but goes beyond it to an understanding of the *personal meaning* of 'illness' for an individual. Individuals interpret illness differently and attach different significances to it depending upon factors such as their past experiences and beliefs and the context in which illness occurs. As speech and language therapists move through their working lives, they understand that no single 'diagnosis' will affect clients in the same way. At its simplest level, the same 'impairment' may be associated with very different outcomes in terms of activity, participation and wellbeing. More fundamentally, communication difficulties can have a significant impact on an individual's sense of identity. For example, Brumfitt has written extensively about the impact of aphasia on the self (e.g., Brumfitt,

---

Box 2.1 Shared decision making

Reflect on a client who you have worked with. Consider how you could implement shared decision making when working with the client. In your reflection, you could consider:

- How will you establish the level of involvement the client wants?
- Who might be involved in the decision making (think about who might be important to the client and how you can explore this, as well as which other professionals will be involved)?
- What are the options available? How can you clearly help the client understand what these are and the evidence for them? Are there any risks? Are there options available? If not, why (for example, lack of evidence for alternative treatment options; predetermined care pathway).
- What are the client's values and goals? Do you have any prior knowledge of the client that can help you to understand these? How can you explore them further?
- Think about your own values and preferences and whether these have (or should have) any influence in the decision-making process.

1993; 1998). Teenagers or adults who have stammered most of their lives may have an identity as 'a person who stammers' which is difficult to relinquish and can make change difficult. Crichton-Smith summarizes this perfectly:

> "Adults who stammer present a unique challenge to the speech and language therapist because, as adults, they have invested years in developing their character but, as people who stammer, they want to change."
>
> *Crichton-Smith, 2002, p.348*

In the context of therapy for stammering, Manning (2010) discusses client factors that influence clinical change, including their 'stage of change', for example, whether they are in a 'contemplation' or 'action stage' and coping style (use of emotion-focused or problem-focused coping styles). Both of these variables are discussed further in Chapters 3 and 4.

Individuals who are diagnosed with an illness or sustain an injury develop *illness perceptions* through which they make sense of their illness or injury (Cameron & Leventhal, 2003). These cognitive models can include beliefs about what they think it is, what caused it, how long it will last, what its consequences will be and whether it can be cured. Negative illness perceptions tend to be associated with poorer recovery and increased use of healthcare regardless of any objective measures of the severity of difficulties (Petrie & Weinman, 2006). Illness perceptions are explored again in Chapter 4.

Within the psychotherapeutic literature, the 'patient as person' has been explored in terms of client characteristics. Certain characteristics, particularly higher levels of expectancy and hope, are seen as an 'extra-therapeutic' or common factor that is influential in change, regardless of the treatment (Grencavage & Norcross, 1990; Lambert, 1992). Although rather removed from the practice of counselling or speech and language therapy, a thought-provoking study in the field of acupuncture illustrates the influence of positive expectations on outcomes (Rosén et al., 2016). The study is particularly interesting because it uses a sham-controlled randomized trial design and a large number of participants. Two hundred and forty-three healthy volunteers were randomly assigned to genuine or sham acupuncture treatment. Within each of those groups, participants were further randomized to 'positive' or 'neutral' communication conditions in relation to expected treatment effect. In the positive communication condition, the therapist conveyed positive statements such as "I have had positive effects on relaxation with this treatment before" or referred generally to studies about relaxation effects. In the neutral communication condition, therapists used statements such as "During treatment, you will just lie down and rest and I will not talk to you much" or referred to the effects of acupuncture on relaxation being uncertain (Rosén et al., 2016, p.4). The study showed that there were no differences in perceived relaxation between genuine and sham acupuncture or between the positive and neutral communication groups. However, although the positive communication style did increase the treatment expectations of participants more than the neutral communication group, there was no difference in perceived relaxation between these two groups. Rather, participants with higher levels of expectancy *before* intervention were more likely to perceive greater relaxation. Hence the authors suggest that "baseline beliefs had a larger impact on treatment outcomes than experimentally induced verbal conditions" (Rosén et al., 2016, p.8). In other words, it was the characteristics of the client – in this case, expectancy – that appeared to influence outcome.

One final point to note here is that gaining an understanding of what a communication difficulty *means* for an individual may not always be straightforward precisely because of the nature of the difficulty. Resources such as Blob Trees (e.g., Wilson & Long, 2009), Visual Analogue Self-Esteem Scale (Brumfitt & Sheeran, 2010) and Drawing the Ideal Self (Moran, 2012) can be a useful way of gaining insight into the personal meanings of communication difficulties for individuals.

The therapeutic alliance

The therapeutic alliance (also often referred to as the 'working alliance' or 'therapeutic relationship', although there are some differences in the way the terms are used) represents a move away from the technical and procedural components of treatment and well beyond the idea that a 'good' health professional-client relationship has value in terms of mediating positive outcomes from management decisions (Mead & Bower, 2000, p.1090). The therapeutic alliance is based upon developments in psychotherapy, particularly the work of Carl Rogers in 1967 who proposed that the 'core conditions' provided by the therapist of empathy, congruence and unconditional positive regard are both necessary and sufficient to bring about therapeutic change in client. A growing body of literature has considered the 'power' of the therapeutic alliance in both counselling and health interventions, striving to 'unpick' the mechanisms that contribute to bringing about change. Bordin (1979) was influential in identifying three components of the therapeutic or working alliance: the 'task' or actual therapy activities, and the client's belief that they are relevant and will work; agreement on goals; and the personal bond between the professional and the client.

A large body of research has focused on the contribution of the relationship between clients and counselling and health professionals, and its contribution to therapy and health outcomes and suggests that the quality of the relationship is a strong predictor of therapy outcomes. Pomerantz (2014, p.264) notes that, in counselling psychology, the quality of the therapeutic relationship seems to be important no matter how much emphasis the therapist him or herself puts upon it. Behaviourists, for example, tend to de-emphasize the therapeutic alliance, humanists emphasize it and cognitive behavioural therapists would fall somewhere in between. Nevertheless, the relationship is essential in the eyes of the client. This is interesting for the speech and language therapist to reflect upon since it suggests that it is not only client groups and 'difficulties' such as voice and stammering, which have traditionally had a strong element of counselling, for which the therapeutic alliance is important. Again in the field of psychotherapy, Wampold (2015) describes a particular common factors model, referred to as the contextual model, which identifies 'the real relationship' is a key pathway in therapeutic change. It is a special kind of social relationship in that it is confidential (within certain limits such as safeguarding issues) and where revealing difficulties does not disrupt the relationship. Taylor (2008) writes in a similar vein from the perspective of occupational therapy; the therapeutic relationship provides a safe place where clients can address emotions and coping. Wampold (2015) also notes that, before therapy can begin, the initial therapeutic relationship needs to be established. He reflects upon research suggesting that humans make very rapid decisions about each other in terms of qualities such as trustworthiness, and suggests that clients are highly likely to engage in the same processes based, for example, on the dress of the therapist and other features of the setting. He also notes that more clients terminate therapy after the initial session than at any other point (Connell et al., 2006).

Box 2.2 Establishing a therapeutic relationship

What contributes to establishing a therapeutic relationship when you first encounter a client? Reflecting on the suggestion that clients may make very rapid decisions about trustworthiness, what factors, apart from what you do or say, might contribute to their decision?

The therapeutic alliance has been explored in the context of both physiotherapy and occupational therapy practice. For example, Morrison and Smith (2013) describe a process in which there was an interpersonal connection between occupational therapists and their clients, derived from the OT's characteristics of being warm and caring, which deepened over time. This provided clients with the 'impetus' to achieve functional improvements which, in turn, led to a sense of success and increased self-efficacy and built trust in the alliance. Palmadottir (2006) interviewed clients about their experiences of occupational therapy whilst in rehabilitation. These findings are interesting because they are relatively unusual in describing examples of participants who did *not* have their needs met through the relationship with their therapist. Their dimensions of 'detachment' and 'rejection' were characterized by a lack of interest on the part of the therapist and, in the latter case, a negative attitude towards the client:

"She often spoke to me as I was a little kid. One is of course confused these first weeks and sometimes when I was shaving myself I forgot to turn off the water and she would say with disdain; well, did we forget something...people that put themselves on a pedestal...maybe she felt her job was so important that she was too good to talk to patients."

Palmadottir, 2006, p.938

In another example, one participant described how the OT put pressure on him to 'take more action and power' when his preference was for the therapist to retain power and be more directive, echoing earlier discussions concerning the importance of identifying clients' preferences for involvement and responsibility.

Besley, Kayes, and McPherson (2011) reviewed the literature on assessing therapeutic relationships in physiotherapy and identified eight key themes: *patient expectations* (of both physiotherapy and outcomes); *personalized therapy*, particularly a holistic approach; *partnership*, including trust; *congruence* between the therapist and patient regarding diagnosis, treatment and goals; *communication*, particularly nonverbal communication and active listening skills; *relational aspects* of friendliness, warmth, empathy, caring and "faith that the physiotherapist believes in the patient" (p.88); *influencing factors* such as the process and environment for appointments and the skills and competence of the therapist; and the *physiotherapist roles and responsibilities*. This final theme related to the role of the therapist in activating the patient's own resources acting as a motivator and, in particular, as educators. In an interesting empirical study, focus groups with physiotherapists in Norway identified three roles; that of educator, partner (relating to the therapeutic relationship) and coach (Solvang & Fougner, 2016). As educators of patients for self-management, "*the best patients to work with are those who embrace the therapist's message, show a willingness both to change behaviour through self-training and to use trial and error to acquire skills and finally, who understand that they must challenge themselves*" (Solvang & Fougner, 2016, p.594). Physiotherapists in the study saw themselves as trying to bring clients around to this way of thinking, "enthusiastically encouraging them" to engage in self-management strategies that have been shown to be effective (p.598). The authors question, however, whether physiotherapists are supportive and respectful of those clients who do *not* fit this profile. Hence, as was seen both in the OT study above and in discussions of shared power and responsibility, there may be a tension between the dominant narrative of patient engagement and empowerment and being patient-centred. When this happens, the relationship with the client is likely to be adversely affected.

Within speech and language therapy, there has been some exploration of the 'role' of the therapist through examining the discourse of therapeutic interactions (Ferguson & Armstrong, 2004; Leahy, 2004; Wilkinson, 2004). Simmons-Mackie and Damico (2011) describe two recognizable types of therapy interaction; clinician/adult teacher-centred therapy and client/child-centred therapy. Within clinician-centred therapy, a typical sequence in the 'request – response – evaluation' sequence (RRE):

> Therapist request: "What is this?" (shows picture of a dog)
>
> Client response: "Dog"
>
> Therapist evaluation: "Good"

Simmons-Mackie and Damico argue that this type of interaction, and others like them, serve to emphasize the asymmetry of the therapist–client relationship in which the therapist has assumed the role of 'judge'. They describe other roles that are 'co-constructed' by participants in the relationship. For example, by using phrases such as "I know you're having trouble with your talking" and "We're going to do some work to help you with your talking", the therapist has assumed the role of 'helper' and the client as 'one who needs help' (p.43).

Fourie, Crowley, and Oliviera (2011) conducted one of the few studies exploring the therapeutic relationship from the perspective of children. They conducted semi-structured interviews with children, aged 5–12 years, about their speech and language therapy experiences. Themes included the therapist as a source of fun, power differentials, role confusion and the physical characteristics of the therapist. Merrick and Roulstone (2011) used a range of supported conversation methods to gather the views of 7–10-year-olds about speech and language therapy. Echoing Fourie et al. (2011) as well as Simmons-Mackie and Damico (2011), they also identified power imbalance, describing a 'discourse of impairment', in which the therapist–child relationship is unequal, with the therapist being perceived as an authority figure and therapy as 'work'. Leahy (2004) has suggested that this asymmetrical therapeutic discourse might be ameliorated through emphasizing the social relationship in interactions with clients, focusing upon the client him or herself, rather than the problem. Plexico, Manning, and DiLollo (2010) offer helpful reflections on actions that might be used to achieve this, for example, following the conversational lead of the client, using summarizing as a way of recognizing the importance of what is said by them and using requests rather than directions in behavioural therapy approaches.

Shill (1979) discussed the role of the psychological aspects of treatment, specifically motivation, when working with clients with aphasia. She discusses the potential value of the patient-therapist relationship in providing motivational 'climate' alongside the specific 'content' of speech and language therapy work, quoting Darley:

> "The clinician therapist continually provides information, insight, encouragement, and optimistic effort; he assuages tendencies to self-criticism, self-punishment, anxiety and despair. By his supportive, non-provocative manner and his systematic schedule of language stimulation he conveys to the patient that the problem is understood and can be dealt with constructively ... this [activity of the therapist] is an essential ingredient of the clinical situation and perhaps in some cases the only one that makes a great deal of difference."
>
> *Darley, 1975, cited in Shill, 1979, p.511*

She calls for research to assess the influence of the relationship on the outcomes of aphasia therapy. Surprisingly, in the intervening 40 years there have been relatively few studies in speech and language therapy which investigate the therapeutic relationship and therapist qualities in any context at all.

The health professional as person

Finally, within their framework, Mead and Bower (2000) consider the role of the personal qualities of the doctor in person-centeredness, a factor very closely intertwined with the therapeutic alliance discussed above. They refer to Balint's concept of 'one-person medicine' in which the aim is to provide a satisfactory clinical description of the presenting 'problem' with no consideration of the doctor her or himself. This is contrasted with 'two-person medicine' in which the health professional is an integral part of the description and there is a recognition that the professional and the patient or client are constantly influencing each other, for better or worse.

The psychotherapeutic literature suggests that between 6 and 9% of variance in clinical outcome is accounted for by individual clinicians. Ebert and Kohnert (2010)) note that individual therapist effects are rarely included in published research but used data published from a study by Rvachew and Nowack (2001) to analyze the difference between the effectiveness of five clinicians delivering treatment for speech sound disorders in children. Their analysis suggested that 20% of the difference in treatment outcomes was accounted for by differences among the five clinicians, regardless of which treatment was being delivered.

In speech and language therapy, there has been some research into the qualities of what we might call 'therapist as person'. Fourie (2009) used interviews with 11 adults who had speech difficulties to explore the therapeutic relationship in speech and language therapy. He used grounded theory to generate his theory of 'Restorative Poise' (Figure 2.1). Therapeutic qualities identified were being *understanding*, *gracious*, *erudite* and *inspiring* (Fourie,

Restorative Poise	
Therapeutic qualities being:	**Therapeutic actions being:**
Understanding Responding to alienation by being patient, interesting, caring, compassionate, really listening	Confident Taking charge and being truthful, frank, open, self-assured, self-possessed, committed, energetic and enthusiastic
Gracious Being courteous, nice, respectful, socially skilled, kind, benevolent, generous	Soothing Being relaxing, reassuring, calming, peaceful, non-threatening, non-defensive, non-punative
Erudite Being knowledgeable, intelligent, educated, resourceful, facilitating reflection, helping to visualize and set goals and re-evaluating of the self	Practical Being relevant, flexible, effective, efficient, helpful, useful, on the right level
Inspiring Being enthusiastic, motivational, arousing clients with stimulating information	Empowering Re-establish autonomy, reconstructing confidence, providing choices, righting upset power balances

Figure 2.1 Restorative Poise (Fourie, 2009, p.989). Reproduced with permission of Taylor and Francis Ltd.

2009, p.989). Therapeutic actions are being *confident, soothing, practical* and *empowering* (p.989). Presented with these findings, many of us may feel daunted and experience a degree of uncertainty in our ability to deliver such noble qualities and actions. Nevertheless, Restorative Poise elucidates how these qualities and actions can be demonstrated (Figure 2.1).

Plexico et al. (2010) explored the perceptions of clients who stutter about the characteristics of SLPs who are and are not effective in promoting successful change. Their findings have many resonances with those of Fourie. Effective clinicians are passionate and committed (in Restorative Poise nomenclature, they are inspiring and confident). They believe in the therapeutic process and the client's ability to accomplish therapeutic change and encourage agentic behaviour on the part of the client (they are empowering). They actively listen, with a patient, caring demeanour (being understanding and gracious) and understand the nature of the problem and its treatment (they are practical). Ineffective clinicians, on the other hand, are seen as judgemental, lacking interest, knowledge or understanding of the problem (they are neither erudite nor soothing) and tend to focus on activities rather than the person (Plexico et al., 2010, p.347). Both Fourie and Plexico frame their studies in the context of the therapeutic alliance, illustrating the close association between the alliance and the personal qualities of the therapist.

Whilst distinct from the idea of 'therapeutic qualities' described above, Baggs (2013) reported an interesting study in which he used the Keirsey Temperament Sorter (KTS) II (http://www.keirsey.com/) to assess the personality types of 320 student speech-language pathologists from six universities in the United States. The KTS is based on Jungian theory and identifies 16 psychological types along the axes of sensing-intuiting (S-I); thinking-feeling (T-F) and judging-perceiving (J-P) as well as an attitude of extraversion or introversion (E-I) (http://www.personalitypage.com/four-prefs.html). Although they found all 16 personality types in their participants, over 50% were ESFJ or ISFJ, twice the proportion expected compared to the US population (Baggs, 2013, p.4). These results need to be treated with some caution but do provide useful points for reflection. Firstly, as Baggs (2013) notes, just because this is the *prevailing* personality type for an SLP/SLT does not imply that this is the *best* personality type for the profession. Baggs discusses the implications of his findings both for the working team and for student education. For example, team members who score highly on perceiving, preferring flexibility and spontaneity may be a source of friction for team members who score highly on judging, preferring planning and order. For educators of prospective speech and language therapists,

Box 2.3 You as a therapist

1. Reflect on therapeutic qualities described by clients in the studies outlined above. Which ones do you see in yourself? Are there any that you would like to develop? Are there any that seem irrelevant or even undesirable? Where are the overlaps and differences between 'you as a therapist' and 'you as a person'?

2. The Keirsey Temperament Sorter is available to do online: http://www.keirsey.com/sorter/register.aspx. Try it and take note of the results. What do you think are some of the implications for those you work with (clients and colleagues)?

there is obviously a need to be aware of learning style preferences. Supporting students and team members to use, for example, a Myers-Briggs assessment to identify their own personality type and that of their peers and colleagues can be a positive step in helping them to understand themselves and others.

Common factors for therapeutic change

So far in this chapter we have explored the relationship between health professionals and clients through the concept of person-centred care, making use of Mead and Bower's conceptual framework to discuss some of the elements that contribute to it. Whilst Mead and Bower's framework has its origins firmly in the 'doctor–patient' relationship, we have extended these discussions to encompass some ideas from wider areas of practice. Three of the dimensions identified within the framework – 'therapeutic alliance' and the interrelated ideas of 'doctor/therapist-as-person' and 'client-as-person' – have strong resonances within the counselling literature as important elements in the *common factors model*. The idea was first mooted by Rosenzweig (1936), citing Lewis Carroll's 'Dodo Bird Verdict' following a race (everyone has won and all must have prizes) as a metaphor for the idea that, whilst many bona fide therapeutic interventions are effective compared to no treatment, no one specific intervention is more effective than another when they are compared against each other (Luborsky, Singer, & Luborsky, 1975).

The dodo bird verdict is described succinctly by Wampold (2001) in relation to psychotherapy. He refers to "a common core of curative processes" (p.ix); a model describes the idea that, whilst many different ingredients, protocols and techniques can lead to successful therapeutic outcomes, the *qualities of the clinician* are essential. Lambert and Bergin (1994) argued that *therapeutic relationship* accounts for 30 percent of change, with 40 percent being external factors (positive or negative) and 15 percent due to expectancy or placebo. Only 15 percent of change in therapy was attributable to technique. More recent analyses, though arriving at different figures, have drawn similar conclusions. For example, Wampold et al. (2002) found that 7 percent of variability in treatment outcomes was due to therapeutic alliance, 1 percent due to specific treatment and 70 percent due to therapists' belief in the effectiveness of treatment.

Common factors can and do encompass not only clinician qualities but also technical skills and behaviours on the part of the therapist. Lambert and Ogles' (2004) 3-stage sequential model of common factors is:

- Support factors (therapeutic alliance, warmth, acceptance, trust, similar to the 'core conditions' identified by Carl Rogers)

- Learning factors (changing expectations/thought patterns)

- Action factors (e.g., practising and mastering new behaviours, facing fears, problem solving).

Grencavage and Norcross (1990) reviewed 50 publications in the psychotherapeutic literature to identify the most frequently proposed common factors. They identified 35 factors in total, categorizing these into five main groups. The first of these is *client characteristics*, particularly positive expectancy and hope. *Therapist qualities* included general 'beneficial qualities' as well as the therapist's ability to promote positive expectancies and hope and warmth and positive regard. Thirdly, a wide variety of *processes of change* are described. These included 'catharsis', or the act of sharing the problem in a safe environment, 'trying something out' and providing a rationale, for example, naming the problem, providing an explanation and putting forward a plausible plan for resolving it. Grencavage and Norcross argue that it is these change processes that, more than any other category, bridge the gap between specific techniques and 'global theories' (Grencavage & Norcross, 1990, p.377). The category of *treatment structure* included the use of the techniques and an exploration of emotional issues as well as frequency of treatment. Finally, *therapeutic relationship* is referred to, particularly the therapeutic alliance, as discussed above.

Common factors in speech and language therapy

There is evidence from a number of clinical areas within speech and language therapy that, whilst studies which compare treatment with no treatment find that treatment is effective with a large effect size, those that compare one treatment with another find a very small effect size. In other words, it is important to do *something* but may be less important to do one particular thing or another. Interesting examples to illustrate this point have been discussed in the literature on effectiveness of stammering therapy. Two reviews of stammering interventions (Nye et al., 2013; Baxter et al., 2015), both identified that there is very limited evidence that one treatment is more effective than the other and refer to the possible influence of common factors, including the characteristics of participants and clinicians, in treatment effectiveness. Similarly, de Sonneville-Koedoot, Bouwmans, Franken, and Stolk (2015) compared direct (Lidcombe) and indirect (based on Demands and Capacities) treatment of preschool children who stammer and found that both treatments were equally likely to reduce stuttering after 18 months. The authors discuss the possibility that common components, such as 1-1 parent-child time, as well as therapeutic alliance, may have a larger influence on outcomes than unique components of therapy. The work of Susan Michie and colleagues, discussed in more detail in Chapter 5, may well be able to make a significant contribution to our understanding of evidence-based practice (EBP) here. Michie's work on behaviour change techniques has provided a framework by which we can 'unpick' each component of a particular therapy approach, with the potential to manipulate it and identify the active ingredient(s). Nevertheless, whilst such work has the potential to result in what might be described as highly 'manualized' therapeutic interventions, the 'art' of the therapist in working with the client to bring about change cannot be ignored. Indeed, as has already been discussed, therapists may matter at least as much - and maybe more - than therapies in determining therapy outcome. Some therapists may feel uncomfortable with this idea and some may even see it as 'anti-scientific' or 'anti-evidence-based practice'. However, a more helpful approach is to see it as a factor that is worthy of much more exploration in intervention research than is currently the case.

There have been extensive discussions of the common factors model and its relationship to evidence-based practice within the psychotherapeutic literature. In an influential paper, Laska et al. (2014) argued for "expanding the lens of evidence based practice". They draw a helpful distinction between 'empirically supported treatments' (ESTs), by which they mean treatments that have proved effective in clinical trials, and evidence-based practice. Referring to the familiar 'triad' of EBP, they emphasize the importance of 'clinician expertise' and 'client preference' and argue for elevating the importance of those factors in understanding and investigating therapeutic change.

Although written some time ago, Ratner (2006) produced a wide-ranging and still highly relevant discussion of the application of evidence-based practice within speech and language therapy in which she reflects explicitly on the role of common factors and the interaction of client, therapist and therapy in bringing about therapeutic effect. Ratner cites Messer (2004) to sum up the difference between medical models of empirically supported treatments (ESTs) and contextual or 'common factor' models:

> "The medical model on which ESTs are based says, 'Seek a therapist who uses techniques with demonstrated ability to alleviate your condition,' whereas the contextual model advises, 'Seek an interpersonally competent therapist who uses a treatment approach that you find compatible with your worldview.'"
> *Messer, 2004, p.582, cited in Bernstein-Ratner, 2006, p.260*

In reality, perhaps one might want to say: "Seek an interpersonally competent therapist who uses techniques with demonstrated ability to alleviate your condition that you find compatible with your worldview." Within this view, it is the interaction between the therapist, the therapy and the client that leads to a successful outcome.

Ebert and Kohnert (2010) investigated common factors by exploring speech and language therapists' beliefs about factors that are most important to effective clinicians. Their first study used interviews to explore the beliefs of speech and language therapists and speech and language therapy students about factors related to the SLT that impact on the effectiveness of treatment, given the same client and the same intervention programme. Three major interlinking themes emerged. The first of these is *behaviours*, which seemed to be specific to intervention situations but, importantly, *not* to specific interventions. These included factors such as motivating the client, measuring change, engaging in evidence-based practice and communication and collaboration with the client as well as with their family, carers and other professionals. Secondly, *traits* such as creativity, empathy and flexibility were identified. Finally, *acquisitions* referred to knowledge, experience and attitudes that could be acquired by time or effort such as knowledge of the disorder, relevant literature, cultural awareness. Some other professional attitudes were also considered to be acquisitions because they can be learned or developed. These included professional motivation, expectations about the client's success and taking the viewpoint of the client (Ebert & Kohnert, 2010, p.138), all ideas that have arisen earlier in this chapter. Ebert later discussed the importance of investigating the extent to which client-clinician relationships influence treatment progress and outcomes in speech and language therapy (Ebert, 2017). She reported on the development of a clinician-client relationship scale, adapted from counselling psychology, designed to gather data from three different perspectives: children having speech and language therapy, their caregivers, and the speech and language therapist. Scales such as this may have important clinical and research applications. For example, they might be used to facilitate patient-centred care by providing a means of gathering feedback about how clients and their families are experiencing the relationship with their speech and language therapist. In a research context, they may provide a way of investigating statistically whether and how the clinician-client relationship - a 'common factor' - influences speech and language therapy outcomes.

The role of expectation and hope

Therapists, including speech and language therapists, provide hope that things will improve. As Pomerantz (2014) insightfully points out, the power of hope will not be lost on anyone who has ever taken their car into the garage and been met by a mechanic who confidently imparts the notion that they can diagnose and repair the problem. Earlier in the chapter, we discussed an acupuncture study by Rosén and colleagues which found that 'baseline' expectancy – in other words, the characteristics of the client – seemed to be more responsible for outcomes than the acupuncturist creating positive expectancy through the communication used during the session (Rosén et al., 2016). However, other studies have found that 'augmented communication', which enhanced the therapeutic relationship, did have a positive effect on treatment outcomes. For example, in another acupuncture study with patients who have Irritable Bowel Syndrome, using questions about how the patient understood the cause and meaning of the condition, expressing empathy and the communication of positive expectancy (through, for example, referring to previous success with using the acupuncture with this client group) resulted in better outcomes than sham acupuncture alone (Kaptchuk et al., 2008). Similarly, in the context

---

Box 2.4 Creating positive expectancy

Janet is Mum to Calum who is 2:9 years old. Calum has significant speech sound difficulties and is mostly unintelligible, even to family members. He is becoming increasingly frustrated. Mum is very keen that Calum needs to 'speak clearly' and wants therapy to start as soon as possible. The SLT believes that auditory discrimination would be the best initial approach to therapy. What challenges might there be for the therapist in developing a positive therapeutic alliance with Mum? How could the SLT communicate positive expectancy? You might find it helpful to think about:

- Expressing empathy with Mum
- Exploring Mum's beliefs about Calum's speech difficulties
- Providing an explanation for his difficulties and linking this clearly to your choice of therapy approach.

---

of psychotherapy, Wampold (2015) argues for the importance of clients believing the explanation provided for their difficulty is coherent and that the treatment approach to be taken will be helpful, as outlined in Grencavage and Norcross's notion of 'catharsis'. Clients and therapists need to agree about both the goals and tasks of therapy and the client needs to believe that therapy tasks will be helpful in coping with his or her difficulties and achieving those goals. These factors are, in turn, vital for developing a successful therapeutic alliance. In Chapter 4, the idea of 'illness perceptions' is discussed, that is, the beliefs that people hold about their difficulties such as what caused them and how long they will last. Exploring illness perceptions may be an important element that contributes to expectation and, hence, the therapeutic alliance, since understanding the client's perspective can inform the way in which the therapist's explanations are accepted by the client.

Influences on person-centred care

Mead and Bower hypothesize a large number of variables that can influence the five dimensions of person-centred care and these are illustrated in their model (Figure 2.2).

Mead and Bower point out that the influences identified are largely hypothesized rather than empirically evidenced and that some influences

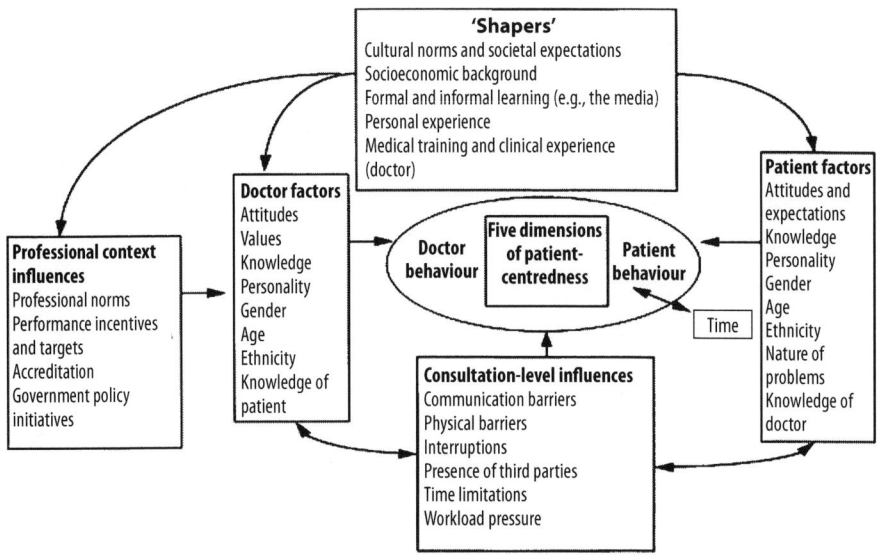

Figure 2.2 Influences of person-centred care.

may be more modifiable than others. For example, as we saw earlier, 'sharing power and responsibility' has been considerably influenced in recent times by policies such as patient choice and self-management. In contrast 'doctor (health professional)-as-person' may be less amenable to change. For some individuals, some aspects of "person-centeredness may require a limited though considerable change in personality" (Balint, 1964, p.121, cited in Mead & Bower, 2000). For speech and language therapists, the role of reflective practice has the potential to enhance their 'therapeutic qualities' and become insightful practitioners with their individual clients and they may find it useful to use Mead and Bower's model as a prompt for thinking about the factors that can enhance or detract from their therapeutic relationships with their clients and person-centred practice. Below, however, we consider in a little more depth two features of contemporary practice that have potential to influence the therapist–client relationship: working in a culturally diverse society and the increasing influence of technology.

Working in a culturally diverse society

Marshall (2000) points out that the large majority of speech and language therapy students in the UK are from the dominant culture, that is, white, Judeo-Christian, monolingual and middleclass. At the same time, it is often the case that limited focus is put on cultural issues in most pre-registration courses; there may be some input on working with bilingual families and perhaps information about certain ethnic minority groups.

Differences in culture can affect the way that people communicate, access social support, and their expectations of and responses to, healthcare professionals and so consideration is important to building effective therapeutic relationships and engaging in person-centred care. Cultural differences have often been understood in terms of collectivism versus individualism. Collectivist cultures, such as those in East Asia or Latin America, may be more likely to place emphasis on attending to others, fitting in and having a harmonious relationship with others compared with more individualistic cultures, leading to the prediction that people from collectivist societies will be more likely to be able to benefit from social support (Shavitt et al., 2016). Further distinctions have been made in terms of collectivist cultures; horizontal societies are more likely to emphasize attachment to their nuclear and extended families, to emphasize sociability in their relationships and to judge powerful others, including health professionals, in terms of compassion and warmth (Shavitt et al., 2016, pp.959–960). On the other hand, vertical collectivist societies place more value on hierarchy and status. Social relationships tend to de-emphasize autonomy and place value on fulfilling obligations and behaving in a way that is appropriate to relative social standing. Asian cultures also seem to emphasize norms that encourage controlling emotional expressions (Ruby et al., 2012, cited in Shavitt et al., 2016). As an illustration of these points, there was racial/ethnic variation on factors that patients consider to be 'very important' when making a decision about surgery from breast cancer, with over 30% of Asian patients rating 'to do what family wanted' compared to around 12% of whites (Hawley & Morris, 2017). Clients from some racial and ethnic groups may favour a medical model and view the SLT as a medical professional. They may, for example, prefer health professionals to 'tell them what to do' rather than engage in shared decision making and may have an expectation that, in paediatric settings, the SLT will work in isolation with the child on their speech, language and communication difficulties (Verdon, Wong, & McLeod, 2016). However, as we saw earlier in this chapter, the desire to be engaged varies on an individual basis (Watts Pappas et al., 2016) and cannot be automatically attributed to any particular differences in culture. Some very basic considerations might include being aware:

- Of the possible different meanings of social support for different cultures. For examples, some cultures may have natural access to wide social support. Others may be reluctant to seek social support because it leads to feelings of obligation.
- That people from some cultural backgrounds may be less willing to discuss holistic needs and implications with the SLT.
- That clients from collectivist backgrounds may be more likely to want to engage their family on decision-making processes.

Bellon-Harn and Garrett (2008) describe a useful model of cultural responsiveness, VISION, for speech-language pathologists working in family partnerships (Figure 2.3):

Values and belief systems: Bellon-Harn and Garrett suggest ways in which the professional might explore their own values, including engaging with the ways in which minority cultures relate to the majority culture, reading material about the dominant culture to understand power differentials and racism and observing media coverage of different cultures and reflecting on the accuracy of representations (p.142). Using

Components of the VISION model	
V	Values and belief systems of the family and professional
I	Interpretation
S	Structuring the relationship between the professional and the family
I	Interactions style of verbal and nonverbal communication of family and professional
O	Operational strategies for accomplishing determined expectations and goals
N	Needs (perceived) by family and professional

Figure 2.3 The VISION model of cultural responsiveness (Bellon-Harn & Garrett, 2008). Reproduced with permission of SAGE/ Hammill Institute on Disabilities. .

open-ended questions can help professionals to understand the values and beliefs of families.

Interpretation: Different cultures' view of the people–nature relationship can influence the way they respond to health professionals. For example, some may believe that they should not interfere with the natural order of things and this may influence the degree to which they want services or are active participants within them (p.143).

Structuring relationships: This component refers to allowing the family to decide who should be included in the clinical process and the degree of family participation (p.144).

Interaction style: Professionals need to be aware of the ways in which cultural influences may affect how individuals respond to nonverbal communication behaviours such as eye contact, physical distance and hand-shaking. Other factors to consider include the use of humour and preferences for written or oral communication (p.145).

Operational strategies: This dimension is concerned with selecting and addressing goals. The authors suggest that speech and language therapists ask, "Why?" questions to interrogate their own values when suggesting the setting goals, for example, "*Why is it necessary for the family to use the device during dinnertime for choice making?*" (Bellon-Harn & Garrett, 2008, p.146). In addition, individuals from some cultures may appear to agree with a treatment plan because of a desire to avoid conflict yet choose not to participate because the plan is not acceptable to them (p.146).

Needs (perceived): Here, the therapist gains insight into what the family perceives their needs to be by asking the question about their hopes for their child, relative or themselves. It is important, then, to show how the therapy goals selected will help the client to reach their long-term outcomes (p.147).

One of the challenges of cultural sensitivity is to understand different cultural groups without stereotyping them. Interpretations and categories of culture are often fluid, complex and transnational (Stewart, 2002) so accurate interpretation of the context is needed and individual difference is still likely to be more important. The idea of 'cultural humility' is described by Tervalon and Murray-Garcia (1998). Rather than 'acquiring a body of knowledge' about the characteristics of various groups, as might be expected with 'cultural

---

Box 2.5 Cultural humility

What are the cultural influences on your own values and belief systems? Remember that these influences might come from your ethnicity, socioeconomic or educational background, religion, gender, age or generation (e.g., Baby Boomer; Generation X; Millennial).

---

competency', it is the ability to continually reflect upon potential biases that may be unconsciously applied in practice with communities, and to recognize that the dominant approach is not necessarily the right approach (Verdon et al., 2016). Cultural humility involves setting aside the SLT's 'expert' status and to recognize that the client has knowledge and understanding that is beyond the scope of the professional through their own personal biography and preferences. Robertson (2007) describes how the building blocks of emotional intelligence – a trait that is often well developed in speech and language therapists – can make an important contribution to working with people whose cultures are different to our own; using the skills of self-awareness, self-management, social awareness and relationship management can make an important contribution to the cultural sensitivity and client-centred practice.

The impact of technology on relationships with clients

For more than 20 years, the internet has provided individuals with information about their 'health'. Clients now have access to much of the same material as professionals and often take this information with them to appointments. There are a variety of reasons why clients might access information, such as to check 'symptoms' in order to diagnose themselves or others, to try and deal with things themselves and to inform a decision as to whether they need to seek professional input at all. If they do decide to seek professional help, they may subsequently seek further internet information following the meeting in order to find out more, to validate what they have been told or, possibly, because they are dissatisfied with what they have been told (McMullan, 2006), essentially seeking a 'second opinion'.

A few studies have explored how the availability and use of internet information might impact upon the relationship between clients and professionals, though it has to be said that the large majority of these focus on doctors. From the point of view of 'the provider', there may be concerns that clients will be unwilling to accept what they have been told or offered, leading to feelings that their authority is being questioned, or that the information that they have obtained is inaccurate. This, in turn, may have a negative effect on the client–provider relationship (Bylund et al., 2007). There is some evidence to suggest that younger or less experienced health professionals may feel more negatively about clients bringing internet information to appointments, perhaps because they feel that they are being tested or have concerns that the client will bring something of which they have limited or no knowledge. For the client, there may be a feeling that the provider disapproves of their internet information-seeking efforts and they may feel reluctant to bring it up during appointments. They may use face-saving strategies such as framing the information they have accessed in terms of direct or indirect questions such as, "What do you think about…" or "I'm worried about…" in order to preserve their relationship with the health professional (Bylund et al., 2007; Dedding, van Doorn, Winkler, & Reis, 2011).

In her narrative review, McMullan (2006) notes that the availability of internet information sits alongside the shift of 'patient' from passive recipient to active consumer of health information, although it has also been suggested that having an interest in acquiring knowledge does not necessarily equate with clients wishing to be actively involved in decision making (Gerber & Eiser, 2001). It is worth noting that, in the years since the review was published, this conceptualization has moved far further with recognition of the 'expert patient' as a valued source of knowledge about their health condition and how best to manage it, as discussed earlier in the chapter. Indeed, the use of internet sources by clients with chronic, long-term conditions may well be seen in a more positive light by health professionals since reliable sources have potential to make a contribution to self-care. Nevertheless, for the speech and language therapist working in a clinic whose (possibly new) client comes to see them for an appointment, reflecting on the different possible response outlined in McMullan's paper (2006, p.27) is a potentially useful starting point:

1. The professional responds defensively. He or she may feel threatened and seeks to reassert his or her authority and steer the client towards a course of action determined by them.

2. The health professional seeks to collaborate with the client. There is recognition that the client may have the time and the motivation to seek new information that they themselves may lack and the balance of 'information ownership' is shifted towards the client. However, there is

also acknowledgement that questions arising from internet information obtained by clients can have a negative impact on the timing of sessions.

3. The health professional engages in 'internet prescription' (Gerber & Eiser, 2001) by recommending websites that are a source of reliable and up-to-date information. The professionals may also provide advice about how to filter information.

It seems likely that many speech and language therapists would be comfortable with a combination of the second and third scenarios – as, indeed, is suggested by McMullan herself. A review of literature on the impact of internet information of physician–patient relationships concluded that enabling clients to share their internet was actually one of the key mechanisms by which healthcare professionals could demonstrate that the opinions of the client are valued, thereby enhancing the relationship (Tan & Goonawardene, 2017).

Where more difficulties might arise are situations in which clients are not simply seeking information about the condition but using internet information to make a case for – or even to demand – a particular type or amount of therapy which may be inappropriate or unavailable in the setting, or to evaluate the choices or performance of the health professional compared with those that they have read about online (Broom, 2005). Some writers have made explicit links between these elements and the rise in consumerism which has "been able to support modern patients in defining, asserting and achieving increased expectations and entitlements in health care" (Buetow, Jutel, & Hoare, 2009, p.99), a point similar that of Owens (2015) discussed in Chapter 1. When health professionals do disagree with the information brought to them by clients, it is suggested that the best strategy is to validate their efforts and/or show the client that they are taking the information seriously (Bylund et al., 2007) in order to preserve the relationship. Buetow, Jutel, and Hoare (2009) discuss the idea of 'role convergence' between health professionals and clients, underpinned by forces such as consumerism and socio-technological changes and conclude that, on balance, it is a positive development.

Aside from the availability of information via the internet, a more recent development has been the use of remote assessment and therapy, usually via video. Telehealth (also known as telepractice and telemedicine) has generated a great deal of interest because it has potential to be an efficient way of delivering services, particularly where large geographical regions are sparsely populated; it may also may offer a promising route to providing specialist services where they are currently limited, as is the case in the United Kingdom for adults who stammer (N. Lieckfeldt, personal communication, May 2017). A number of studies have explored the use of telehealth in different areas of speech and language therapy practice including voice disorders (Kelchner, 2013), dysphagia (Ward et al., 2012), paediatric language difficulties (McDuffie et al., 2016) and stammering (Carey, O'Brian, Lowe, & Onslow, 2014).

In this chapter, we have focused on the relationship between therapist and client and questions naturally arise about whether and how telehealth might impact upon that relationship. A few studies have explored the effect of telehealth on the therapeutic alliance in psychotherapy. Simpson and Reid (2014) reviewed the literature and concluded that, largely, the components of the therapeutic alliance remain present when therapy is delivered by videoconferencing, as reported by both clients and therapists. They found evidence that therapists often make adjustments such as checking with clients for clarification. Interestingly, they note that clients have commented that telehealth can lead to feelings of greater control and personal space which enhances the therapeutic relationship. There was also some initial evidence that clients may be more active in therapy that takes place via video than face-to-face and hypothesize that this may be because they feel a greater sense of ownership and responsibility for their part in the relationship and, perhaps, feel less intimidated and therefore safer to discuss feelings and problems (p.295). These findings are very encouraging in the context of speech and language therapy practice and we hope that the next few years will bring more research exploring clients' experiences as well the effectiveness of speech and language interventions delivered via telehealth.

Ending therapeutic relationships

Much of this chapter has been concerned with the nature and power of therapeutic relationships. The ending of this relationship, through the process of discharging clients, is therefore something that is worthy of careful consideration, both from the perspective of the client and that of the speech and language therapist. In pre-registration education, a great deal of attention is usually paid to the processes of taking a case history, conducting formal and informal assessments, devising an intervention plan and measuring outcomes. Discharge may be considered in the context of the client meeting specific therapy goals, 'plateauing' or, increasingly, having come to the end of an episode or package of care. Very little attention is usually given to the *process* of ending therapy or to the impact that this can potentially have on both parties.

Deborah Hersh has written extensively and thoughtfully on discharge in speech and language therapy. She has interviewed speech and language therapists about their experiences in the context of aphasia therapy (Hersh, 2001, 2003) and written the lead article for a special edition of the *International Journal of Speech-Language Pathology* which focuses on discharge in different speech and language therapy settings (Hersh, 2010). Drawing on literature from psychotherapy, social work and rehabilitation, as well as her own work, Hersh discusses three interwoven tensions that underpin the process of discharge.

Real vs ideal endings

In an ideal world, therapy would end when a client is cured or has reached agreed goals to the satisfaction of both therapist and client. Real endings, on the other hand, are enmeshed within "*complex and varying political, economic and geographic contexts*" (Hersh, 2010, p.288). Such factors might include financial and resource constraints, an emphasis on early discharge, or the need to prioritize specific clients such as those with dysphagia and working within a proscribed organizational framework such as 'assessment and recommendations'. All these factors carry with them the attendant requirement to manage caseloads accordingly. Speech and language therapists interviewed by Hersh often reported that they felt a tension between wanting to carry on supporting their clients, particularly if there were no further services available, and the recognized need to prioritize clients and manage their caseloads effectively. Hersh refers to earlier work which suggests that a mismatch between the realities of providing healthcare and experiences 'on the job' and personal motivations for entering the profession (to help people) are a source of dissatisfaction for speech and language therapists (Byng, Cairns, & Duchan, 2002; Whitehouse, Hird, & Cocks, 2007). Baker (2010) refers to the recurrent disappointment that can be experienced by speech and language therapists when resource constraints result in an inability to provide an optimum service (p.326), potentially leading to a perceived eroding of expertise and poor job satisfaction. Anecdotally, we have found that it is not unusual to meet speech and language therapists who have made a choice to enter the private sector not because they are intrinsically motivated by running a business or making a profit, but because they believe that they will be better able to offer services to clients which are congruent with their personal and professional values of providing ongoing care.

Building and breaking therapeutic relationships

Hersh and a number of others in the 2010 Forum on discharge refer to Coltart (1993) who writes of "*the paradox of building authentic relationships that are destined to be broken*" (p.327). Whilst authenticity is the crux of what makes the relationship powerful, it is also artificial (Hersh, 2010, p.286), predicated on professional provision of time-limited services. Baker (2010) argues that, whereas attention has been paid in the psychotherapeutic literature to the impact of ending therapy on the therapist, the value of the relationship to the speech and language therapist is generally neglected. Because the profession of speech and language therapy is often chosen by individuals who have a disposition for caring for others, there may be a blurring of professional and personal boundaries, leading to feelings of sadness, guilt or loss on the part of the therapist when therapy ends. The power of these feelings for some speech and language therapists is eloquently summed up by the title of Hersh's paper, a quote from one of her interviewees: "I can't sleep at night with discharging this lady…". Thus, the qualities of empathy and caring, powerful tools in the therapeutic alliance, have the potential to lead to attachments which are problematic for both therapist and client.

Hersh has written about speech and language therapists' use of the strategy of 'weaning' clients from aphasia therapy (Hersh, 2003):

> "The practice of weaning (allows SLTs) to achieve their imperative of moving clients on while maintaining the integrity of their therapeutic relationships. In their efforts not to upset, abandon, or reject clients … weaning delayed, softened & obfuscated the harsh reality of leaving the supports of therapy … It involved a rhetoric of negotiation that protected (SLTs') caring image, legitimised their actions & helped hide the inadequacies of provision for people with chronic aphasia."
>
> *Hersh, 2003, p.1026*

We reflect further on the emotional impact of working as a healthcare professional in Chapter 4.

Promoting client empowerment versus professional control

Finally, Hersh (2010) reflects on the need to balance client empowerment, a strong principle shared by most speech and language therapists, with need to maintain professional control. The need for control is frequently driven by the need to control resources and therapists may be mindful of the possibilities of clients complaining or making unrealistic demands on services although there is little evidence that this happens in reality (Roulstone & Enderby, 2010). Nevertheless, as Owens (2015) argues, the idea of choice, a concept deeply embedded within the notion of client empowerment, is only relevant where there is a meaningful choice – in this case, to continue therapy – to be made.

Strategies for discharge

Practical strategies proposed for managing discharge include:

- Being specific from the outset about goals, policies and packages of care (Roulstone & Enderby, 2010). Management systems such as East Kent Outcome System (Johnson & Elias, 2010) and Malcomess Care Aims (Malcomess, 2005) are examples of frameworks which make such discussion with clients specific. Many speech and language therapy services publish or make explicit their pathways to set expectations from the outset.

- Early involvement of family and friends to foster social engagement within the community to reduce the possibility of over-dependence on the therapist, involving the idea of a 'circle of support' and 'fading support' over time to increase self-reliance (Togher, 2010, p.322).

- Replacement of commissioned speech and langue therapy services with other sources of support such as self-help groups following discharge. Another practical example comes from many pre-registration speech and language therapy courses that run conversation partner schemes where pairs of students visit a person with communication difficulty (often aphasia) providing opportunities for practising communication strategies. Such schemes are often enthusiastically taken up by speech and language therapists discharging their clients as a means of offering further input. Increasingly, there may be the potential for some types of support to be accessed online.

Speech and language therapists need to ensure they engage in self-care, developing awareness of their feelings and discussing them in mentorship or clinical supervision. This is discussed further in Chapter 4.

Conclusions

The focus of this chapter has been on the nature and impact of the relationships that we have with our clients. In doing so, we have drawn widely from literature across the professions, particularly that of medicine and psychotherapy, but also from other allied health professions as well as from speech and language therapy itself, using Mead and Bower's conceptual framework of person-centred care as a way of organizing themes and ideas. Whilst there are many approaches to understanding the relationships that health or other professionals have with clients, many common themes emerge, with perhaps the most fundamental of these being the power of the relationship itself.

3 Personal and social change across the lifespan

Introduction

There is always a risk that the personal context of the individual with a communication difficulty can be overlooked when intervention decisions are taken, because of the need to focus on evidence-based management of the impairment. Yet the individual's background and life experience may be critical to clinical outcome. Taking a person-centred approach involves an understanding of the individual's social context, with knowledge and understanding about how personal growth and change takes place over time. Understanding these different psychosocial aspects helps to identify factors which may influence the individual's experience of a communication difficulty and this in turn may influence the response to speech and language therapy intervention. Personal and social development is multifaceted, influenced by development in cognition and biological processes as well as social and personal experiences from infancy to old age. These influencing factors may be both internal (cognitive and biological processes) and external (psychosocial changes). In this chapter, the focus is on the latter.

Box 3.1 Personal and social change

When Graham had to cope with his stammer in his teenage years this coincided with his personal transition to adulthood. He faced challenges about his general self-image and also to his educational progress resulting in issues of low self-esteem and low confidence which were in addition to the feelings he had about stammering. But when he reached late middle age, his views and attitudes were different. He had many family and work-related responsibilities which allowed him to consider his stammering in relation to those roles and permitted a more reflective and considered view of the impact of his speech on his everyday life.

We know that social development involves the way an individual's interactions and social relationships grow, change or remain stable over the course of life. What is also of interest are the consistent characteristics that differentiate one person from another and how these change within individuals. For some individuals, development may be a smooth process with occasional disruptions from relatively typical social and cultural changes, such as moving from single to married status. But for others, development may be difficult from the start; a child with a significant speech and language delay may have a less trouble-free experience than a child who has no obvious challenges. Clegg, Hollis, Mawhood, & Rutter (2005) studied 17 men with severe receptive developmental language disorders (DLD) at four time points (9.11y; 13.04y; 24.03y; 36.03y). They were compared to non-language-disordered siblings and an IQ matched comparison group. At the mid-30 age time point the DLD cohort had significantly worse social adaptation including long-term unemployment, limited close friendships and limited romantic relationships. Joffe, Beverly and Scott (2011) report the experiences of young people who have grown up with a speech and language difficulty and quote one individual's experience as being "a real kind of overwhelming kind of challenge sometime" (p.123). The implications for this individual are that the challenges of coping with a developmental communication impairment have impacted upon social and educational development over time, interacting with challenges in everyday life.

This chapter focuses on the processes of ageing, reviewing frameworks that help us to understand the ageing process and considering how these processes might interact with having a disability.

Theoretical frameworks for understanding psychosocial development

Assumptions relating to the age of the individual need to take into account the variations in personal and social maturity. Thus, one adolescent may have mature social attitudes and cope well and another may be less socially able and struggle to cope in spite of the fact they are both the same age. Age ranges in social and personal development should therefore be construed as averages rather than exact scales. In order to consider the role of psychosocial development, three theories will be considered, each of which make an important contribution to our understanding of the processes of ageing. The three theories are, in many ways, complementary as they offer insight into how an individual moves through the ageing process from infancy to old age, the contextual and systemic factors that influence human development and the way in which challenges encountered over the lifespan can lead to personal growth or decay.

Erikson's Psychosocial Theory of Development

The researcher and author Erik Erikson greatly influenced the understanding of the psychosocial stages through which an individual moves during the lifespan. Erikson (1968) described a set of eight stages to explain individual experience and development. These stages provide an explanation for how the individual grows and develops and how the different stages finally culminate in the experience of old age.

Infancy (0–1 year): Basic trust versus mistrust. During the first stage, infants are attempting to make sense of their worlds. Reliance on a consistent and stable caregiver is critical to the successful transition from this infancy stage to early childhood. If the relationship with the caregiver provides for the core needs of the infant this is considered to form the foundation for future successful relationships.

Early childhood (1–3 years): Autonomy versus shame. The child is developing independence through the discovery of skills and abilities such as putting on clothes and shoes, or playing with toys. According to Erikson, parents must allow their child to explore the limits of their abilities, enabling them to develop a sense of independence and confidence within the safety of the family.

Play age (3–6 years): Initiative versus guilt. By the time the child has reached this stage there should be successful development of interpersonal abilities, using opportunities for planning activities and initiating new ideas. Erikson argues that if the child is limited in attempts to play freely through negative feedback from caregivers, the child will develop a sense of guilt and discomfort and be likely to lack self-initiative in the future.

School age (aged –12 years): Industry versus inferiority. Children will be learning to read and write, to do maths and to be creative. The role of the teacher becomes important in the child's development. Similarly, the child's peer group may gain significance, influencing self-esteem and the child's motivation to win approval. Erikson notes concerns that if the child does not feel approval from their parents or teachers this may affect the child's future potential.

Adolescence (12-19 years): Identity versus confusion. The child has reached a stage in which future adult roles are being developed through new experiences and reflections on identity. The child needs to develop a sense of self and identity which becomes consistent over time. This includes different components of the self, such as body image, academic and occupational, and sexual. If a consistent sense of self is not developed then this may lead to role confusion,

Early adulthood (20-25 years): Intimacy versus isolation. Individuals are likely to develop closer relationships with others, such as longer-term commitment with someone other than a family member. If this stage is achieved successfully it will allow the young adult to experience comfortable relationships with a sense of safety and care. Those young adults who avoid relationships and fear commitment can experience future isolation, loneliness and depression.

Adulthood (40-65 years): Generativity versus stagnation. According to Erikson, during middle adulthood careers are established, individuals settle down within a relationship, possibly begin their own families and develop a stronger sense of being a part of society. If none of these objectives are achieved, Erikson described the individual as feeling unproductive and unhappy. Clearly, since the development of these ideas, the objectives which Erikson has described as desirable may have changed within the values of society today.

Old age (65 years-end of life): Integrity versus despair. Productivity, as a general rule, slows down and individuals start to explore life as a retired person. Although retirement age has changed since Erikson described these changes, and there may be different expectations about growing older, in general the notion that elderly individuals review their lives and reflect on achievements and losses still stands. If the elderly individual cannot see their life in the context of a meaningful integrity the individual is more likely to be prone to a sense of hopelessness and depression. According to Erikson, successful integration as an elderly person leads to wisdom.

Although Erikson's theories are descriptive and developed during the 1960s, one of the strengths of the framework is that it provides an explanation for psychosocial development right across the lifespan, using not just the individual's personal and internal developmental components, but also the social and contextual factors that are influential. Whilst contemporary readers may reflect that the nature of these social and contextual influences has changed significantly since Erikson developed his theory and may also dispute the chronological ages identified within each stage, the processes described by Erikson nevertheless continue to be relevant in understanding human lifespan development. For the speech and language therapist, an awareness of these processes can illuminate our understanding.

Ecological Systems Theory

Whilst Erikson's theory takes into account the role of social and cultural influences on human psychosocial development, the framework described by Urie Bronfenbrenner takes this further. As its name suggests, Bronfenbrenner's Ecological Systems Theory views the individual's development as being systematically influenced by everything in the environment. The Ecological approach suggests that different environmental levels simultaneously influence individual development. Bronfenbrenner (1979) describes five major levels which account for how the individual is influenced over time at different stages in the lifespan. Thus, the different systems may overlap and form multidimensional components of individual experience. The everyday immediate environment including interactions with parents/caregivers, siblings, neighbours, colleagues, teachers and so on is described as the microsystem. Links between elements of the microsystem environment are seen in the mesosystem. Much broader environmental influences are seen in the exosystem, which refers to the experience of the individual's community contexts. This is considered still linked to the individual's personal circumstances. For example, a parent may work in the community and their rota, place of work and the type of work may have a direct impact upon the child's experience. Thus, both the micro- and mesosystems are embedded within the exosystem. Greater cultural influences, such as the type of society, ruling government context and religious systems will also affect the child and this is referred to by Bronfenbrenner as the macrosystem. Children in families who move from one culture to another (refugees, for example) are likely to be strongly affected by this system and the macrosystem is likely to be different for different generations. For example, there is an emerging acknowledgement that further research is needed on the development of children in refugee camps who have been impacted by war. The American Psychological Association (2010) has reported on this. Finally, the chronosystem – which refers to timing in relation to development – is also influential. Here, the child's experience will be affected by *when* events occur.

According to Bronfenbrenner (1979) significant life events will have a more significant developmental impact on the younger child compared to an older adolescent or adult. For example, a bereavement at age 3 will have a different impact to a bereavement in adulthood.

Box 3.2 Ecological Systems Theory

Spend some time drawing your own ecological system. With yourself at the centre, add the direct influences on you in the first layer (microsystem), followed by the wider context (exosystem) and, finally, the broader cultural context (macrosystem). You can also add arrows to represent links between the micro- and exosystems (the mesosystem). Reflect on the role of digital technology and social media in each layer of Bronfenbrenner's Ecological System. Think about similarities and differences between your experiences (particularly the macrosystem) and the possible experiences of an individual who is (a) quite a lot younger than you and (b) quite a lot older than you.

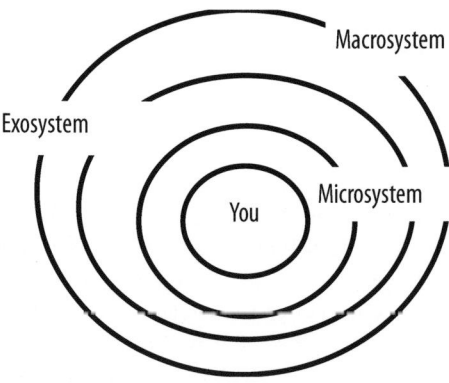

Lifespan Model of Developmental Challenge

A more recent approach to understanding lifespan development is found in the Lifespan Model of Developmental Challenge (Hendry & Kloep, 2002) which describes the core concepts of resources and challenges. Hendry and Kloep's (2002) position is that age is not relevant in the model of human development because resources, challenges and risks are the influencing factors. They argue that each child is born with potential resources and challenges in their lives, and throughout development these will have an impact on the individual's experience. Resources and challenges are classed as features of physical, cognitive, emotional, social, material and environmental development and will vary across individuals. Thus, whenever an individual is facing a challenge, the system of resources versus the specific challenge will influence outcome. Kloep, Hendry and Saunders (2009) give the example of a female child who, because of her gender, may not be encouraged to play in a boisterous manner. Arguably, this child will develop fewer resources in the form of self-defence, leaving her more vulnerable to the risk of assault and leading to potential effects on self-efficacy and health status. According to Kloep et al. (2009), these resources reflect those aspects of micro- and macrosystems (Bronfenbrenner, 1979) where individuals' resources are influenced by such societal issues as family circumstances, healthcare opportunities, employment or cultural factors.

Another example of how resources could operate is that of a child born with sporting potential who may develop high-level sporting abilities if they have strong guidance from a mentor who allows the child to develop new skills and increase self-confidence. Alternatively, another child may have the same sporting potential but not receive good guidance, so that their capacity to achieve well in the sporting context is diminished. This construct may also be applied to the child with a developmental communication impairment. If the child is in receipt of good therapeutic and educational support along with strong family support, the child may develop good coping skills over time. However, if these support systems are not in place, then the child will have less capacity for coping over the lifespan and the challenges faced become a serious risk to successful development.

For children in extreme situations, such as those caught up in wars, the risks and challenges will be very acute and potentially life changing. Refugee children, for example, may have been exposed to personal injury or observed injury and killing of their own family members. A report by the American Psychological Association (http://www.apa.org/pi/families/refugees.aspx)

identifies many risks for children covering the impact of sexual and physical abuse and the emotional and physical consequences, along with traumatic brain injury and physical scarring from severe wounds. All of these conditions will affect emotional and cognitive functioning over time. In terms of developmental challenges, the specific issues are whether a refugee child has the resources to cope with the challenges from these conditions, ranging from internal personal factors to whether there are available social and structural supportive resources from within the community they are placed in.

The system of challenges facing an individual across the lifespan may enable the individual to build on capacities or alternatively not respond well to the challenge and perhaps ignore or try to avoid coping with a challenge. It is this feature which Hendry and Kloep (2009) believe discriminates between individuals. If an individual is ultimately able to respond to and cope with a particular challenge, then the individual's resources are increased and strengthened. This amounts to developmental growth occurring. However, if the individual is unable to cope with a challenge (i.e., there is a mismatch between tasks and resources), their resources will be diminished and 'decay' will occur in the sense that the individual may fail to develop and progress or cope with the challenge.

The model of developmental challenge described by Kloep and Hendry (2009) can usefully be applied to the healthcare context. In the model they demonstrate that the individual copes with life 'tasks' on the basis of the resources available to them and in relation to the severity of the challenges they face. Clients may face challenges such as coping with education, work or family commitments when they (or their family member) are facing illness or disability. The model provides a framework through which to consider the client in the light of the individual resources available to respond to a challenge and, crucially, how these might be developed so that the individual can successfully meet the challenge.

Each of the three theories outlined above has the potential to enhance speech and language therapy practice. Erikson's description of 'stages' can support our understanding of the ways in which a communication or swallowing difficulty might interact with, or even disrupt, the developmental processes that an individual is experiencing, whilst Ecological Systems Theory encourages the speech and language therapist to look beyond the individual and their immediate family to explicitly consider the broader context of the exo- and macrosystems that influence development. Finally, the Developmental Challenge model offers a framework for considering the interaction of resources and challenges faced by individuals as a result of, and beyond, the difficulties that brought them to speech and language therapy. Nevertheless, the theories offer little in the way of discussion of disability and, in the remainder of this chapter, the focus is shifted onto more explicit consideration of how disability can affect individuals across the lifespan.

Box 3.3 Developmental challenge

Jason is 2:6 years old. He is using few words and sometimes tries to make himself understood by pointing and vocalising. Mum is quite good at predicting what he needs and tries to avoid tantrums by doing this as much as possible. He is very active and likes to run around. Sometimes he can appear aggressive, biting or punching things and once or twice he has kicked his Mum.

Jason's Mum, Sally, lives with Jason and his younger brother, Nathan, who is 1 year old. The boys' Dad moved out of the house just after Nathan was born. Sally works part time in the local supermarket and her Mum helps her out with the boys, though this is getting increasingly difficult because Sally's stepdad has cancer and her Mum feel that she should be spending more time with him. Sally's stepdad finds it hard to be around the boys, particularly Nathan, because they are quite boisterous.

Following assessment, you have identified significant delay in Jason's language development. Your view is that a child–parent interaction approach would be beneficial for Jason and his Mum.

Thinking about the 'developmental challenge' perspective:

What 'tasks' can you identify that Sally needs to meet?

> Sally has a number of 'tasks' or challenges: Within the past year, she has experienced a significant change in her family circumstances with the birth of a second child and her long-term relationship has broken down. Sally is now the mother of two young children, one of whom currently has some additional needs in relation to his communication and behaviour. She is juggling single parenthood with work and it may be that financial resources are stretched. Another family member has a serious illness. There are likely to be physical and emotional challenges associated with this; Sally has to cope more on her own as her Mum is less available meaning that, between working and looking after the boys, she probably has limited time for herself and feels tired. She is likely to be worried about her stepdad and there may be other feelings, such as guilt at placing additional demands on her Mum and not being able to help her in the way she would like.

continues

What role do you think the proposed intervention might play in the developmental challenge model? How might it be viewed by Sally?

Interventions such as parent–child interaction require time and commitment from parents, with attendance at regular appointments and strategies and activities to practise in between. In addition, Sally has been trying to avoid tantrums by predicting Jason's needs and therefore strategies to develop his communication may, in the short term, mean that his frustration increases. Engaging in therapy at this point may be viewed by Sally as another 'task demand' that adds to all those she is already experiencing. Sally may already feel insecure and anxious if her 'resource pool' is low in comparison with the demands she is facing, and attending therapy and implementing strategies might be viewed as a further drain on the pool. When there are multiple concurrent challenges, there is a risk that 'decay' could occur, with a downward spiral of drained resources leading to Sally feeling overwhelmed and unable to cope because of the mismatch between demands and resources.

How could the SLT try and minimize the 'risk' arising from a mismatch between 'tasks' and 'resources'? In particular, think about (1) How you could identify resources that Sally may already have, and (2) How you can develop skills that will be helpful in meeting the tasks.

There is evidence that Sally already has some good coping resources. Although we only know a small part of the picture in terms of demands and resources, she has been able to attend a clinic appointment, an achievement which should not be underestimated, and she clearly knows Jason well. It would be important for the SLT to explore with Sally the skills and resources that she already has. One way of doing this might be to use tools from Solution Focused Brief Therapy (see Chapter 6) such as coping questions and past success questions. On a practical level, the SLT can work with Sally to identify the explicit physical resources – time and place – where communication strategies can be implemented; these need to be realistic. Rather than making suggestions immediately, it would be preferable to ask Sally about her 'typical day' so that the ideas can 'fit in' and require minimal additional resources. The SLT may be able to provide advice about behaviour management or refer to another professional. Self-efficacy is an important resource (see Chapter 5). The SLT can support increased self-efficacy by ensuring that Sally experiences success with activities (setting appropriate targets). A group approach to intervention may be helpful because it offers opportunity to learn from others as well as the potential for social support. Maximizing resources in this way should increase the likelihood that Sally will avoid developmental decay and will develop coping resources which can be drawn upon in future challenges.

Disability and development across the lifespan

Disability, as a term, includes a wide range of conditions and aetiologies. Generally, we distinguish between disability occurring from the developing foetus and at birth, such as cerebral palsy, and disability occurring as the result of an illness or accident which may affect a person at any time in their lifespan (Bogart, 2014), such as a teenager involved in a serious road traffic accident and being left with significant mobility challenges. There are also differences in disabilities where the condition can be seen, such as someone with mobility problems who uses a wheelchair, and another person who may have a learning or communication disability which cannot be visually identified. Perception of visually obvious and hidden conditions may be treated differently by society. Thus, integrating the disability alongside an understanding of psychosocial factors across the lifespan is complex. Indeed, many researchers who aim to explain the factors affecting development across the lifespan have not included the impact on lifespan development when the individual has specific disabilities to manage. This is noted by Smart (2012) who provides a useful discussion and description of disability across the lifespan, noting that progression over the course of the lifespan tends to be viewed in terms of positivity (marriage, graduation, birth of a child) as opposed to negative life events which are generally not seen as part of a transition but more as an individual aspect for which society has more limited means for acknowledging.

Other ways of considering the issues associated with congenital and acquired disability relate to the sense of self and identity, particularly the degree to which individuals incorporate the disability into their self-concept. Olkin (1999) discusses the view that the sense of self or self-concept which embodies the disability is strongly influenced by social group identity. In particular, the negative aspects of disability are socially constructed through social stigma and 'the disabled' can be perceived as a minority group. In turn, this impacts upon the individual's self-concept which incorporates difference and minority into the sense of self. If the influence of society is powerful, then a child growing up with a congenital disability may develop a stronger sense of the disabled self than the individual with an acquired disability who has experienced a loss of function. On the other hand, in the case of a congenital disability, the individual may adapt well over time compared with the individual with an acquired disability (such as loss of mobility) who may continually rely on the memories of past self and therefore experience psychological discomfort. The differences between the two populations are not well understood and more work needs to be done so that we can understand this better (Bogart, 2014).

Box 3.4 The experience of acquired disability

Harry is a 66-year-old male who had his first stroke three years ago resulting in occasional word-finding difficulties. Harry worked in the building trade for 40 years and, according to his daughter, "lived and breathed work". Eight months ago, H had a further stroke resulting in severe dysarthria and dysphagia. Harry lives independently but family relations are fraught. Harry feels his family infringe on his independence. His family worry that he is at risk because he refuses to accept help. They feel that Harry has not accepted his disabilities. Harry is socially withdrawn and expresses embarrassment because his communication is largely restricted to gesture and facial expression and he has poor saliva control. Initial SLT input was aimed at improving function through oromotor exercises. Harry worked diligently at these, practising every day. At a 6-month review, there were no changes to speech and swallowing function. Further input would consider compensatory forms of communication. Harry refused to use the AAC device or to attend a 'Total Communication' group offered by the SLT service. He was therefore discharged from the service.

Why might Harry be refusing the intervention offered by the SLT?

The vignette suggests that Harry may still be in a phase of assimilation following his second stroke. He appeared to be very engaged in speech and language therapy when it was aimed at restoring his previous communication and swallowing function but this has changed now that the focus has shifted onto using alternative communication strategies. Harry's difficulties from his first stroke were relatively mild and this may contribute to a continued belief that he will make further progress with his speech and swallowing although the evidence suggests that this is not the case. The broader picture also needs to be considered; for example, Harry may be experiencing low mood or depression. It is possible that Harry may benefit from psychological intervention to support adjustment to his changed self. He may be more able to engage with speech and language therapy at a later time.

Biographical disruption

In terms of developmental challenges facing the individual over time, other researchers have looked for an explanation of what happens when significant challenges have to be faced, such as in serious health events.

One particularly useful framework for understanding how individuals change following a significant health event can be found in the field of sociology. Bury (1991) developed a framework to look at the concept of chronic illness and the potential change to the self. In a very well-recognized body of work, Bury developed the concept of 'biographical disruption' when considering the impact of a health condition on the individual's sense of self. Bury describes two types of 'meaning' in chronic illness: that of the consequences upon the individual from the impact of disruptive symptoms and, secondly, the personal significance of the condition. The individual may have to face the social understanding of the condition along with their own internal perceptions about what the condition means to them. Charmaz (2002) postulated that the self is disrupted by the experience of chronic illness but her data also showed there may be a tendency for individuals to resist reconstructing an altered perception of self around illness as a way of psychological protection. This suggests that it is psychologically 'safer' to retain the old sense of self than risk the challenges involved in creating a new post-illness identity. A further potential way of viewing this is through identity process theory (e.g., Whitbourne, 1986; Sneed & Whitbourne, 2003). Although the theory is focused primarily on ageing, it can also provide a useful way of understanding an individual's response to an acquired disability. It describes a dynamic equilibrium between the established cognitive and affective schema held by an individual about him- or herself and the *experiences* of that individual, for example, the process of ageing or acquiring a disability. In the *assimilation* phase, evidence that challenges an individual's self-concept or schema is dismissed in order to maintain 'self-consistency'. Clients in this phase may, for example, talk about returning to their old job even though this may not be realistic, and may be reluctant to engage in activities that challenge their old sense of self (joining a group, for example). At the same time, this results in the person having limited or no opportunity to engage in experiences that could lead to *accommodation*, whereby the individual adapts their existing self-concept.

An example from the literature on stroke highlights some of these points. In a five-year follow-up study of individuals with stroke, Pallesen (2014) explored how each individual managed their life with stroke. Following analysis of in-depth interviews, the main themes about self and identity showed that, after five years, individuals saw themselves as 'not ill' but as someone with certain disabilities. They felt different from others but recognized that they had to relate differently to their lives post-stroke and, finally, that they had become an individual who had more limited opportunities now than before the stroke, particularly in relation to their social selves. Viewed through the lens of identity process theory, the individuals in this study seem to have undergone a process of accommodation.

Developmental challenge in children

Although developmental stages in the growth of the child are widely described, the specific impact on development in atypical situations is less well understood. Erikson's (1968) early psychosocial stages acknowledge the significance of successful transitions at each stage and, in Erikson's framework, the challenges faced in difficult circumstances may have a negative effect upon overall development across the lifespan. Similarly, developmental stages in the growth of the child will be affected if the child is born with a significant disability. Depending on the nature of the disability, these components may be affected in a variety of ways. Learning disability, for example, will impact across all areas of biological, social and psychological development. Being born with dyslexia may not necessarily impact upon biological development but has potential to impact upon psychological and social development.

In the early stages of the life of a child whose development is not typical, parents may be involved in the stage of seeking a diagnosis for their child's difficulties and often the diagnosis may be devastating news for the family. Psychologists refer to the parents' assumption that their child will be their ideal child, and when a disability is found then they may respond to this as they would do to a significant loss. It is important to recognize that, when a disabled child is an infant, he or she may seem very similar to their siblings and friends, but as they start to grow the discrepancy between a child who is disabled and a child who is not becomes larger and more obvious, confronting the parents and family with increased feelings of loss and grief (Smart, 2012).

Smart's account of the ways in which developmental stages are affected by disability provides a useful framework for the work of a speech and language therapist. Notably, Smart states that the developmental stage at the time of onset or diagnosis will have an important impact upon the individual's response (see Bronfenbrenner, 1979). In addition, the way in which an individual progresses through different stages of their life course will be affected by the type and extent of their disability along with the level of support they have. She notes that there is little positive social role guidance for children with disabilities. However, understanding for children and adults with disability has improved with the raising of awareness through the media, educational inclusion and the Equalities Act (2010).

Developmental challenge in children with communication difficulties

---

Box 3.5 The young child with communication difficulties

Josh started school at age 4 and showed some nonfluent episodes in his speech along with some phonological difficulties. His parents are concerned that he might develop a stammer. He had attended nursery and although his confidence has improved he remains a sensitive boy, for example preferring to play with just one friend at school and not mix in groups at playtime.

What issues need to be considered in relation to Josh's overall development?

Josh is beginning school with communication difficulties along with some concerns about his avoidance of mixing with a lot of children. In order to develop comfortably in the school setting Josh may need help with his communication and also further support in managing in the classroom setting. Although at age 4 it is difficult to predict the long-term impact of his difficulties, it would be important for professionals and parents to have an awareness and strategy for management.

Children who have developmental speech and language difficulties experience a range of challenges in their early and subsequent later years when managing at school. ICAN (Factsheet A: www.ican.org.uk) refers to the potential challenges a child may face in a school setting. Although not all children will experience this degree of challenge it is important to note that these issues have all emerged in some form across the population of children with speech and language difficulties. They include literacy difficulties, difficulties accessing the curriculum and therefore achieving in school, social isolation, disaffection and boredom, behaviour problems, bullying, and low self-esteem (www.ican.org.uk).

Snowling et al. (2006) examined 71 young people with a preschool history of speech-language impairment at ages 15–16 years using a psychiatric interview, questionnaires and parental reports of behaviour and attention. The psychosocial adjustment results were compared to age-matched controls. The children whose difficulties had resolved by 5.5 years had a good outcome, but the outcome was less good for those children whose difficulties persisted, with raised incidence of attention and social difficulties. Thus, for children with specific communication difficulties the speech and language therapist needs to take into account the broad base of potential challenges that may need to be faced as the child is growing up and making transitions through the stages of personal development. This impact should not be overlooked.

Developmental challenges in adolescence

Adolescence is an important part of the human lifespan, linking childhood to early adulthood. There are specific risk factors for the adolescent relating to physical health and mental health. According to Erikson (1968), the key conflict at this stage in the lifespan is identity versus confusion and, to an extent, this is confirmed by later authors. Santrock (2001) describes adolescence as being in two parts: the Early stage, which includes most of the changes arising from puberty and transition from junior school, involving biological, cognitive, and socio-emotional changes; and the Late stage, which involves the latter half of the second decade of life and is defined by career interests, mixing with lots of people of similar age, going out on 'dates' and the process of identity exploration.

Lyn Turkstra has written extensively in the impact of communication impairments and cognitive impairments in adolescents, mostly with acquired neurological disorders but also including autistic spectrum condition (ASC) and specific language impairments. According to Turkstra (2000), adolescence can be seen in the context of three stages. Preadolescent (9–12 years) includes a period of rapid physical growth, the development of independent values and opinions, inconsistent abstract reasoning, the need for privacy, and to be an 'insider' in a group. The early adolescent phase (13–16 years) includes the development of secondary sexual characteristics and sexual behaviours with a focus on physical appearances, a shift to loose, mixed-sex social groups with increased intimacy of individual friendships, and a need for self-reliance, self-appraisal and consideration of the future. Finally, the late adolescent phase (17+

years) is seen as having no specific end point owing to individual variation. This phase includes independent living skills, the continued development of personal identity, morals and values, the inconsistent execution of ideals, high expectations for self-regulation, and the developed responsibility for self-directed learning.

Because adolescence is such a critical period in social development, the risks for individuals who have communication impairments such as ASC, stammering, learning disability or acquired neurological impairments can be considerable. Turkstra and colleagues outline the potential for significant penalties for poor social 'performance' in adolescence including on peer rejection, difficulties with dating, making friends and participating in social activities and maintaining employment (Turkstra, Williams, Tonks, & Frampton, 2008). Furthermore, these penalties have potential to be recursive since social isolation can limit opportunities for social development through practising social skills in peer relationships. Adolescents who have grown up with specific challenges may therefore have difficulty progressing through the adolescence phase.

In a National Longitudinal Study of Adolescent Health, Svetaz, Ireland and Blum (2001) compared differences in emotional wellbeing in adolescents with and without learning disabilities. Of a total of 20,780 adolescents, 1301 were identified as having a learning disability. Following analysis of interview data along with statistical comparison, adolescents with learning disability had twice the risk of emotional distress and females were at twice the risk of attempting suicide and for involvement in violence. So there is clearly some evidence to show that developmental challenges, such as having a learning disability in adolescence, may be exacerbated by many health conditions.

In his own video, Rory Hoy (2006) talks about his experiences of autism and what impact it has on growing up. As an adolescent, his insight has increased but he still has to cope with some of the possible social and interpersonal difficulties. Like many people with autism, he experiences feelings of social confusion, fearing certain situations and experiencing anxiety. He talks about his dislike of physical contact with unfamiliar people and his hypersensitivity in general. His obsessions, particularly challenging in childhood, also mean that his adolescent years are difficult to manage. For teenagers on the autistic spectrum, having an understanding of self and identity is often a challenge. This is well documented and material on adolescence and transition can be found on the National Autistic Society web pages (http://www.autism.org.uk/about-autism/A.aspx).

There may be challenges, too, for adolescents who stammer. In Australia, Erickson and Block (2013) examined self-perceived communication competence and apprehension, stigma and disclosure and experience of teasing and bullying of 36 adolescents who stammered. After analysis, the results showed that adolescents who stammer have below average self-perceived communication competence, heightened communication apprehension, are teased and bullied more than their peers, and try to keep their stammering secret.

There are significant social and personality effects on an individual who has suffered a traumatic brain injury, such as increases in impulsivity, challenging behaviour, irritability, emotional volatility, anxiety and depression, and negative impact upon social relationships. This condition is more commonly seen in adolescents and young adults compared to other age groups. Ylvisaker and Feeney (2000) report that many of these adolescents with TBI will have demonstrated oppositional behaviour prior to their injury. They describe how, when delivering workshops on rehabilitation of adolescents and young adults with brain injury, they use a cartoon of a Doberman dog jumping from a window with the caption, "The Doberman threw himself out of the second-story window soon after he realized the family had indeed named him 'Binky'" (Ylvisaker & Feeney, 2000, p.407). The analogy of 'binkification' describes the idea that typical interventions may attempt to focus on transforming the TBI 'Doberman' individual into a more socially appropriate 'poodle'. However, as Ylvisaker and Feeney (2000) point out, interventions need to take into account the pre-injury personality features of the individual if the approach is to be successful. Simpson, Gale, and Denman (2009a) reported on how they used Ylvisaker's concept of identity mapping when working with an individual with traumatic brain injury. The approach involves the client identifying a metaphorical figure or concept (such as a real or fictional character or an animal) and using this as a basis for forming an identity map with the figure at the centre and characteristics of the figure leading off from this. These could include associations (who would you spend time with; where would you go); feelings (how would you feel to be this sort of person/thing); values (what would be important to you); goals (if you were this sort of person, what would your goals be); and actions (what would this sort of person do to reach their goals). This can then be used as a way of eliciting goals for rehabilitation. Simpson, Gale, and Denman (2009a) describe how their client found the process of identity mapping a valuable and motivating way of organizing his thoughts and "giving direction to his hopes and aspirations" (p.14). In many ways, this process of identity mapping might be viewed as similar to the process and aims of other techniques such as self-characterization used in personal construct psychology or, to a lesser extent, a miracle question as used in solution-focused brief therapy (see Chapter 6); each of these tools provides a means of "understanding people as they understand themselves" (Ylvisaker, McPherson, Kayes, & Pellett, 2008, p.722) as well as eliciting goals that are personally meaningful to them. In their companion piece, Simpson, Gale and Denman (2009b) describe how they have further built on Ylvisaker's ideas by the use of projects within a rehabilitation setting, such as planning a fund-raising event, giving a presentation to a CEN, or producing a self-advocacy DVD when working with clients. This approach can be particularly helpful with clients who have difficulties with executive function or self-regulation such as often occurs with TBI, because it enables the incorporation of client-centred goals and can make use of Ylvisaker's 'Goal-Obstacles-Plan-Do-Review' executive function routine which supports aspects of executive functioning such as planning, initiating, monitoring, evaluating and flexibility (Simpson, Gale, & Denman, 2009b, pp.12-13).

Challenges in adults and middle age

The period of young to middle adulthood is much less researched than childhood, adolescence and ageing. It may be because the group is so large and diverse, making focused research more difficult. Developmental psychologists generally consider early adulthood to range from age 20 to age 40 and middle adulthood to range from 40 to 65. Although there may be much individual variation, in early adulthood one of the primary motivations is that the individual is concerned with developing the ability to share intimacy and seeking to form relationships. At this stage, children may result from long-term relationships. Concurrently, the early adult is often building on work and career decisions which will have long-term effects on socioeconomic status. Interacting with these significant developments will be the development of long-term ethical and moral values, political attitudes and psychological wellbeing. Since the Children and Families Act (2014), support for children and young people with Special Educational Needs and Disabilities (SEND) must now cover the 0-25 age group with plans in place for transition into adulthood. This means that speech and language therapists will increasingly be working with the later years of this age band and therefore need to be cognisant of the younger adult context.

By middle adulthood, the roles that individuals take may diversify and may become more onerous. Individuals may be responsible for their children and extended families. They will have the potential for increased responsibility in the work environment and this may impact on their socioeconomic status and their wellbeing. In relation to Erikson's model the problem posed at this stage is 'generativity versus self-absorption'.

The major tasks which individuals may face in middle age are described by Havighurst (1963) as, firstly, developing acceptance and adjustment to physiological changes such as the menopause. Part of this phase also involves family responsibilities, such as to ageing parents who may need caring for and to teenage children who may need support in order to become responsible adults. The individual may reach and maintain satisfaction in their occupation and will at this time have achieved adult social and civic responsibility. Havighurst also describes the maturation of relationships and exemplifies this as relating to spouse as a person. Clearly, there is the potential for a wide variation in these aspects owing to differing personal circumstances.

Box 3.6 A unexpected challenge in middle age

Jane's third child had left home for university and she was beginning to enjoy more freedom and the chance to do an online literature course. The diagnosis of multiple sclerosis has been very difficult for her to accept and understand, just at this point in her life when she had expected to relax.

How might her personal circumstances and current developmental stage affect the way a therapist approaches any interventions? What would a therapist have to be aware of?

It would be important for the therapist to acknowledge with Jane that her symptoms had developed at a critical point in her life. Time may need to be spent on talking this through. Jane may have to deal with the challenge of strong negative feelings about her loss of abilities and freedom at this stage in her life and may experience anger and sadness. Jane would need to feel engaged with the therapy intervention and the therapist would have to be certain that Jane wanted to undertake the rehabilitative tasks. It may be important for the therapist to support Jane in understanding how the interventions will help her in the future and to enable her to find ways to continue with her literature course and take up other opportunities.

If the middle-aged adult has to respond to the challenge of disability, then it is possible that all of the typical tasks or challenges described by Havighurst may become too difficult or even impossible. For example, the person who has a stroke may find that all of their coping resources have to be focused on recovery and survival. Other roles or tasks, such as caring for growing children or ageing parents, may become difficult or impossible. One way of looking at this can be found from Kloep et al. (2009) who describe developmental transitions as 'normative-social shifts' and more unusual circumstances as 'quasi normative shifts'. Their definitions state that normative shifts include those aspects in society which occur within the framework of the law and the culture. Quasi normative shifts refer to experiences which are not prescribed to the same degree and can be relatively low-level cultural and individual differences, such as fashion, or much more serious and significant changes brought about by accident, illness, moving to another country or radical career change.

During the adult middle years, individuals with communication impairments may include those who have a stroke at a relatively young age, coping with progressive neurological disease, brain injury and maintaining improvement and managing developmental speech and language conditions. These conditions may impact upon the aims and motivation of this age group and the speech and language therapist will need to be alert to these factors.

Challenges for the older person

It is important to consider the impact of ageing upon the individual's personal experience, taking into account the social and personal experiences which may emerge at this time. In order to understand this impact, we need to firstly consider what is involved in the process of ageing and whether the individual's actual numerical age permits us to understand them fully.

Gravell (1988) wrote that, "Ageing is a developmental process which extends throughout life. Ageing causes differences, not deficits, for disease and disorder are not inevitable correlates of old age" (p.1). According to Bromley (1974), chronological age was not necessarily a guide to physical or mental capacity, or even life expectation.

Woodrow (2002) discusses the issues around the definition of ageing and being old. Commonly, distinctions are made between the young-old (65-75), the middle-old (75-85) and the old-old (85 plus). Although in some contexts it may be useful to understand the elderly in this way, it may also be an unhelpful distinction to use because of the wide variation in individual experience. Unlike children's milestones where it is relatively easier to have expectations about phases (expectations about age of walking, speaking and so on), the categorization of the elderly according to age group may be counterproductive as there are less clear-cut assumptions about what changes can take place.

In a very important study, Snowden (2002) examined the experiences of nuns as they grew older. The particular significance of this study is that all of the participants had lived similar lives, been unmarried and had no children, thus creating a study population with a homogeneous lifestyle This well-known 'Nun Study' is a longitudinal examination of ageing and Alzheimer's disease following 678 members of the School Sisters of Notre Dame aged over 75 years. Convent archives were made available to investigators as a resource on the history of participants. The study includes reviews of autobiographical essays by the nuns upon joining the order, administration of memory and cognitive tests to the nuns (some over 100 years of age), tests of physical strength and post-mortem examination of their brains. The autobiographical accounts revealed some highly interesting findings in relation to Alzheimer's disease; sisters who wrote detailed and complex accounts in their youth tended not to develop the disease whereas whose accounts were lacking linguistic complexity were more likely to develop Alzheimer's disease later in life.

We know that there is an interaction between the biological features of ageing and the personal changes that individuals experience as they grow older. Even with an elevated retirement age, the fact of retirement means that many people change their perspective on life and develop a different lifestyle to when they were an employee. Thus the ageing process may be a time of transition, of personal change when perspective on many aspects of life change. Families grow up, they may move away, partners or spouses die, individuals cope with bereavement, ill health, financial changes.

The English Longitudinal Study of Ageing (ELSA) has provided us with a broad and significant understanding of what it means to age in a UK society. Specifically, one study has looked at the self-reported experience of growing older which identified factors influencing levels of exclusion from society. Based on questionnaire and interview data, the study found that the key factors included: age and the increased risk as individuals grow older; family type and whether the individual was isolated in their living circumstances; health, including risk of both mental or physical health conditions; whether the individual had a secure income and ownership of housing; mobility factors such as access to a car; and also access to a telephone. Those individuals with everything in place were less at risk from social exclusion or isolation. Based on one strand of the ELSA data which looked specifically at men (ELSA, 2012–2013), it was found that 1.2 million older men experience a moderate or high degree of social isolation and 0.7 million men experience a high degree of loneliness. The study also reported that men were more isolated than women. These results were achieved by looking in detail at the number of social contacts experienced and reported by research participants and comparing number of contacts with children, other family members and friends between male and female participants.

The potential impact of social isolation is that it brings with it further risks of mental health and depressive difficulties. Family support alone has been shown to be beneficial, but the social networks which are strengthened by friendships are also important (ELSA, 2012-2013; Chopik, 2017). We know that socially active elderly people will use their cognitive skills more frequently than those who are less socially active and that socially integrated lifestyle has been shown to protect against cognitive decline (Fratiglioni, Paillard-Borg, & Winblad, 2014). Figure 3.1 shows the different aspects of ageing and how they might influence the elderly person's experience.

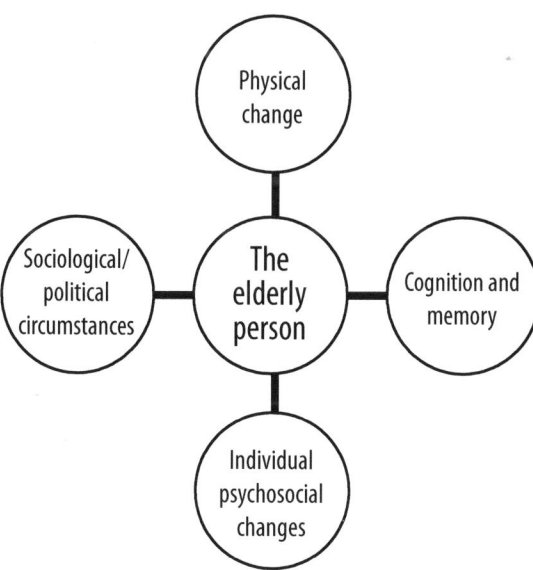

Figure 3.1 Influencing factors in ageing.

Two major theories explain the psychosocial aspects of ageing in older adults. Disengagement theory (Cumming & Henry, 1961) views ageing as a process of mutual withdrawal in which older adults voluntarily slow down by retiring, as expected by society. Supporters of disengagement theory take the view that mutual social withdrawal benefits both individuals and society because it permits the ageing person an opportunity to take less responsibility and allows the younger individual to take more responsibility and mature. Activity theory (Havighurst, 1963), on the other hand, sees a positive correlation between keeping active and ageing well. The supporters of activity theory believe that mutual social withdrawal runs counter to traditional American ideals of activity, energy, and industry. To date, research has not shown either of these models to be superior to the other. In other words, growing old means different things for different people. Individuals who led active lives as young and middle adults will probably remain active as older adults, while those who were less active may become more disengaged as they age. According to Davidson (2002), these views on ageing need to be updated to take account of the changing patterns in society, the different demographics and the variation in attitudes toward ageing. Cultural expectations about ageing are changing rapidly, and with the changes in work patterns and pensions and more diversity in ethnic groups and family groups, the sociological impact of ageing may involve much more variation than has been seen in the latter part of the 20th century.

Erik Erikson (1968), who took a special interest in this final stage of life, concluded that the primary psychosocial task of late adulthood is to maintain ego integrity (holding on to one's sense of wholeness), while avoiding despair (fearing there is too little time to begin a new life course). Those who succeed at this final task also develop wisdom, which includes accepting without major regrets the life that one has lived, as well as the inescapability of death. However, even older adults who achieve a high degree of integrity may feel some despair at this stage as they contemplate their past as it is unlikely that anyone would believe that every aspect of their lives had been perfect. By reviewing their lives, individuals may move towards a more comfortable resolution about how they have lived and what they have experienced.

How do we age successfully?

Life expectancy has increased substantially over the previous century as a result of advances in the way ageing is managed and the medical interventions

Box 3.7 Reflections in old age

Lionel (85 years old) had retired from his job as a laboratory technician in a school and since then has completed a degree with the Open University. He had been a keen sportsman in his youth and had been particularly strong as a runner. When he married and had three children with his wife (Marjory, who died three years ago) he stopped competing in running competitions. On looking back at his life he now considers his decision not to stay in competitive running might have been a bad decision. His life has been enhanced by his close family life and stable job, but his real desire to be a successful sportsman has not been achieved.

available to support individuals as they grow older. Although there is clearly variation across different cultures, in general populations can expect to have a greater life expectancy. For example, there were over half a million people aged 90 and over living in the United Kingdom (UK) in 2014. And for every 100 men aged 90 and over in 2014 there were 249 women (ONS, 2015).

Given these statistics, governments across the world are faced with specific challenges around the needs of the elderly and their social context. Of interest is a report by the World Health Organisation on ageing and health, outlining a framework to foster Healthy Ageing across all cultures (http://www.who.int/ageing/events/world-report-2015-launch/en/). This demonstrates the worldwide recognition that increases in the elderly population mean that all societies will have to consider how they will manage this population in terms of economic factors, health and wellbeing. This issue of how the elderly cope in society was examined by Bowling and Dieppe (2005) who discussed the factors which appear to be influential in achieving a successful old age. These factors relate to biomedical theories and psychosocial aspects. Based on an analysis of current literature they described the main features of successful ageing as: life expectancy; life satisfaction and wellbeing; mental and physical health, cognitive function; personal growth, learning new things; physical health and independent functioning; psychological characteristics and resources; social, community, leisure, participation; social networks and support; accomplishments, enjoyment of diet, financial security, neighbourhood, physical appearance, productivity and contribution to life, sense of humour, sense of purpose, spirituality. These authors also note the importance of asking the individuals who age about their experiences in addition to the broader-based research trials. They note the importance of acknowledging we are still learning about ageing, and need to incorporate not only results from the scientific method but also more qualitative and nuanced understanding.

The very old

According to a report for the Office for National Statistics (2015) the number of centenarians (people aged 100 and over) living in the UK has risen by 72% over the last decade to 14,450 in 2014, with 780 of those estimated to be aged 105 or more, double the number in 2004. England and Wales had more centenarians per 100,000 population in 2014 than Scotland or Northern Ireland. These differences reflect higher life expectancy at older ages in England and Wales compared with Scotland and Northern Ireland. For example in the National Life Tables (2012-2014), at age 85, life expectancy was 5.9 years for males and 6.8 for females in England and Wales. This means that a man aged 85 could expect to live to age 90.9 and a woman to age 91.8. For comparison, the life expectancy in Scotland is 5.5 and 6.4 years, and in Northern Ireland it is 5.7 and 6.6 years.

For our societies, understanding the experience of living beyond 100 years is relatively new territory. Does the individual of 100 years and above merely experience the typical ageing process but it just takes longer than for those who die before they are 100? Or does the experience of being a centenarian mean that lived experience is qualitatively different? In an interesting and original study, Hutnik, Smith and Koch (2012) interviewed 16 centenarians living in the UK and asked them to tell the story of their lives. Based on the content of the interviews, six common experiences emerged. Hutnik et al. (2012) found that all the interviewees had retained strong interests and were the types of people to show resilience in the face of stress. The key themes were: engagement in the world; happiness and describing a good life; stoicism; sources of support; sources of frustration; and talking about death. In these themes, the participants were able to demonstrate the personal capacities which they believed allowed them to live a long life. The role of stoicism is particularly interesting and relates to the more recently-used term in a psychological context, that of resilience (see Chapter 4), seen as an important dimension in the developing child.

Darviri et al. (2009) interviewed nine Greek centenarians of both sexes about their experiences of growing old beyond the age of 100. The qualitative research explored social and life experience and strategies and personality characteristics which influenced the exceptional longevity. Three key themes emerged: social selectivity; conflict avoidance; and adaptiveness. In terms of social selectivity, participants were characterized by their approach to socializing with other people and a clear tendency to avoid conflicts. In addition, these individuals had managed to overcome adversity in their lives and adapt successfully to major life changes, findings similar to those of Hutnik et al. (2012) outlined above. The authors argue that these three themes may be possible pathways to better understand the capacity to age beyond 100.

Ageing in the person with a disability: A developmental challenge

In the same way that the number of elderly people is increasing, the number of people with intellectual disabilities and developmental difficulties is increasing in the ageing population. As with our understanding of centenarians, our understanding of the personal and social experience of people who are ageing with intellectual and physical difficulties is limited. How does the individual with a developmental disability cope with ageing?

There are health risks often specifically associated with certain conditions. People with Down Syndrome are known to be at high risk for a range of age-related health problems including Alzheimer's disease (Lott et al., 2011). Ageing may impact on other longstanding conditions such as ASC, and this has been recently examined in The Autistic Society report on ageing (2013). There are specific challenges for people with autism as they age, such as whether the individual has sufficient insight to be able to recognize their health status. Examples are given of difficulties in recognizing pain and communicating symptoms to care givers. As pain and other health conditions will be more likely to increase as the individual ages, then these challenges will also increase. The report notes that dementia may be difficult to diagnose, particularly the difficulties in distinguishing between communication problems and developing symptoms of dementia. The authors also question whether the condition of autism increases the likelihood of developing dementia. The report concludes that there is insufficient research about ageing in autism. Guidance on ageing in autism can be found through charity websites such as The Autistic Society and Autistica (http://autism.org.uk; http://autistica.org.uk).

In an examination of the experience of getting older for people with learning difficulties and their families, Ward (2010) highlighted the need for services to recognize the specific issues arising when the individual with a learning difficulty grows older and that they may not be able to remain in the family home. In a project entitled 'GOLD: Growing older with a learning disability', Ward talked to many individuals and families about their experiences. The main themes which concerned her participants included the importance of having a home and protection for the ageing person whose parents and caregivers may die or be unable to care for them. In addition, it was found that individuals held strong views about living a fulfilling home life and sought as much independence as possible. Like the elderly person who has no learning disability, the same principle applies to the learning disabled: that of remaining active for as long as possible in order to maintain abilities. Ward (2010) reported the need to invest in planning for the future to ensure that the needs of this population are met and their individual circumstances can be taken into account. It is common for many older people with learning disabilities and their families to be unknown to services until they are in crisis and Ward cautions against this.

The challenge of dementia

Although there are different forms of dementia, the most common form in the elderly is Alzheimers (approximately two-thirds: http://www.alzheimersresearchuk.org/about-dementia/helpful-information/symptoms/). This may develop over several years and is often difficult to diagnose in the early stages. Often the dementia symptoms may resemble symptoms in other conditions. Apathy, for example, may be present in dementia alongside apathy as a symptom in depression. Typical early signs of dementia include forgetting events, names and faces, or repetition occurring as part of everyday behaviour, such as repeating the same question. In addition, losing items or putting them in odd places, confusion about the date or time, getting lost in familiar places, word-finding difficulties and the development of apathy, loss of interest and engagement. As the length of the condition increases, the symptoms become more severe in presentation.

Dementia has therefore emerged as one of society's challenging conditions to manage, particularly because it is increasing across the population. According to Alzheimer's Research UK, there are currently 850,000 people with dementia in the UK (2017), and this number is projected to rise. The impact of dementia will be felt by the individual and the family members and some of the emotional reactions may be complex and challenging to deal with. An individual with early stage dementia may have awareness and understanding and thus feel nervous and confused about the future. The Alzheimer's Society discusses approaches to providing emotional support for people with dementia and for their carers, and note that the confirmation of a diagnosis may trigger depression and anxiety in some people (https://www.alzheimers.org.uk/download/downloads/id/1768/factsheet_depression_and_anxiety.pdf). The Society recommends looking at lifestyle changes which may ease the practical burdens, making use of talking therapies where possible, and also using medication to help individuals cope. There is no doubt that the diagnosis of dementia forms a major challenge for the individual, who may fear the future in terms of everyday activities, access to social care and economic costs. It is one of the sad ironies of the condition that it occurs at the time in the later part of the lifespan when the individual may have less resources to cope with such a huge challenge. Erikson's 'old age' phase of integrity and despair, where the person's capacity to review their life and reach a resolution is viewed as important, may no longer be accessible if the individual develops dementia.

Younger people may also develop early onset dementia (https://www.youngdementiauk.org/) and need substantial support, along with individuals with any type of developmental disability, such as learning disability and autism referred to earlier in the chapter. Young onset (or early onset) dementia refers to people of working age, usually between the ages of 30–65 years. There are more than 42,000 younger people with dementia in the UK, or over 5 percent of all those with dementia (https://www.alzheimers.org.uk/download/downloads/id/1766/factsheet_what_is_young-onset_dementia.pdf). People with a learning disability are at greater risk of developing dementia at a younger age (https://www.youngdementiauk.org/living-learning-disability-and-young-onset-dementia). The Young Dementia UK website reports studies which have shown that one in ten people with a learning disability develop young onset Alzheimer's disease between the ages of 50 to 65. An even greater number of people with Down syndrome develop Alzheimer's disease, with one in 50 developing the condition aged 30–39, one in 10 aged 40–49 and one in three people with Down syndrome predicted to have Alzheimer's in their 50s. One of the key challenges in early onset dementia in people with learning disabilities is the confusion over the diagnosis, when often behavioural symptoms can be mistaken for the learning disability profile rather than attributed to signs of developing dementia. The risk of dementia must therefore be a consideration for the speech and language therapist in certain contexts where people with learning disability are part of the case load.

Box 3.8 Descriptions of ageing

Write down some words which describe ageing from your point of view. Ask a friend to do the same and compare your ideas.

Conclusions

Across the lifespan, individuals are growing and changing in response to their environment, the challenges they face and their personal perceptions and interpretation of their lives. For the speech and language therapist, this contextual background to the communication difficulty may be of importance in understanding how the client responds to therapy. At face value, the individual's background may be relatively hidden, but the therapist needs to have an awareness and sensitivity to the changes and influences a client may experience. Theories of ageing, such as those of Erikson, Bronfenbrenner, and Hendry and Kloep provide a framework through which the speech and language therapist can gain insight into the processes of ageing whilst recognizing that these will be different for each individual. Disabilities, including communication difficulties, and their wider social impact can both influence, and be affected by, the ageing process.

4 Illness and stress: Coping and resilience

Introduction

Health professionals frequently observe that individuals differ in the way they experience and respond to illness. Understanding these different perceptions has the potential to play an important role in working successfully with clients. Chapter 2 discussed the importance of 'patient as person' or 'client characteristics' to person-centred care and building a therapeutic alliance. In this context, the relevance of clients' beliefs about their illnesses or difficulties was briefly considered. In the first section of this chapter, ideas from health psychology about illness perceptions are discussed alongside their application in speech and language therapy. The next section focuses on stress, something that frequently accompanies illness and disability but is also part of all lives, including the working lives of health professionals. Ways of coping and the importance of developing coping resources with our clients and for ourselves are explored. The concept of 'emotional labour' is introduced as a way of understanding the impact that the emotional 'work' that forms part of our everyday professional lives can have. The chapter concludes by building on the idea of coping; some ideas from the field of positive psychology are outlined together with thoughts on how these might be applied in speech and language therapy practice in relation to both our clients and ourselves.

Perceptions of being ill

When individuals, or their children, become ill or have a 'health problem', they tend to develop an organized pattern of belief about their difficulty (Leventhal, Diefenback, & Leventhal, 1992). These illness cognitions, also referred to as illness beliefs or illness perceptions, are an individual's implicit, commonsense beliefs about their condition. Illness perceptions generally fall into five main components:

- **Identity** refers to diagnosis and symptoms. For example, I have laryngitis (diagnosis) with a hoarse voice and sore throat (symptoms).

- **Perceived cause** of the illness. For example, my laryngitis was caused by a cold or my hoarse voice was caused by shouting.

- **Time line**, that is, the perceived timeframe for the development and duration of the illness, e.g., my laryngitis will be over in a few days and my voice will return to normal.

- **Consequences** refers to the perceived effects of the illness which may be long or short term, e.g., my hoarse voice will prevent me teaching which will prevent me going to work. I might lose my job.

- **Curability and controllability** (by self or powerful others), for example, if I follow the advice of the speech and language therapist, my voice will return to normal.

Some theories include additional illness cognitions such as acceptance and benefit finding. Illness cognitions influence the individual's emotional response to illness which, in turn, influences their coping behaviours. This relationship has been described in a number of frameworks variously known as the Illness Perceptions Model, the Illness Representations Model, the Self-Regulatory Model, and the Common-Sense Model of Self-Regulation (CSM). Leventhal's CSM essentially describes three stages: (1) **interpretation** or making sense of the problem; (2) **coping** with the problem; and (3) **appraisal**, or assessing how successful the coping strategy has been (Ogden, 2012, p.221). The notion of patients' coherence (that is, their understanding of the illness) has also been added to the model and this is seen as an important concept in adherence. For example, *if* a client believes that her voice problem is caused by shouting, *then* she is more likely to change her behaviour and stop shouting.

Interpretation

A number of factors are thought to influence the way in which an individual perceives symptoms of illness, including gender, life stage, personality type and coping style (Morrison & Bennett, 2012). Mood, cognition and social context (Ogden, 2012) can also have an impact.

Coping

Ogden (2012) examines coping with illness through Moos and Schaefer's (1984) conceptualization of physical illness as a *crisis*. Changes that contribute to the crisis include changes in role and identity, for example, from independent adult and 'breadwinner' to 'dependent person who is ill'; changes in locations, such as to hospital, and changes in social support, such as isolation from friends and family, and changes in the future (Ogden, 2012, p.232). For example, a young university student may have been looking forward to a future career, having a family and so on that is derailed by a head injury following a moped accident during a summer trip in Europe.

Lutz, Young, Cox, Martz, and Creasy (2011) explored the crisis of stroke through the experience of patients and their family caregivers. They described a trajectory of crisis through three phases, each of which speech and language therapists are likely to be involved in for clients with dysphagia or aphasia:

- **Phase I: The stroke crisis**. In this phase, the patent is admitted to care. They (if they are aware) and their family begin to realize what has happened to them and experience feelings of confusion, loss and fear. Family members may blame each other for not recognizing the symptoms of stroke. At this stage, the patient and family may have limited understanding of the challenges ahead.

- **Phase II: Expectations for recovery**. Once the acute phase is coming to an end, decisions need to be made about future options. Stroke survivors and their families begin to recognize impairments but may also feel hopeful and optimistic. However, many of them still believe that they would stay in rehabilitation until they 'got better'; their definitions of improvement are different from that of the professionals working with them.

- **Phase III: The crisis of discharge**. Although discharge is a highly anticipated event, a further crisis is created when family caregivers realize what adjustments have to be made to accommodate the stroke survivor. Numerous practical questions arise, which seem overwhelming. Once home, stroke survivors realize that they have to depend on others for things that they had taken for granted, leading to feelings of frustration, sadness and grief. Caregivers are worried about caring for the stroke survivor on a daily basis and, in some cases, taking on household responsibilities such as paying bills.

Although based on a small sample, this study paints a vivid picture of the crises that can be faced by individuals and their families following stroke. The role of coping and appraisal are discussed further below in relation to stress (for example, problem-focused versus emotion-focused coping) but are equally relevant here.

Appraisal

Appraisal refers to the way in which the individual evaluates his or her approach to coping. If the coping strategy is effective, the person is more likely to continue to use it.

The relevance of illness perceptions

The illness perceptions of individuals influence their coping patterns (e.g., Leventhal, Safer, & Panagis, 1983), psychological wellbeing (Hagger & Orbell, 2003), medication adherence (Horne & Weinman, 2002), and quality of life (Foxwell, Morley, & Frizelle, 2013). For example, if a client with chronic dysphonia has different beliefs about the cause and controllability of their voice problem (e.g., a disease, and in the SLT's control) to that of the SLT (e.g., psychogenic or behaviour-related and within the client's control), this is likely to be detrimental to important aspects of therapy such as developing a therapeutic alliance and adhering to treatment. Buck, Drinnan, Wilson, and Barnard (2007) explored the illness perceptions of people with dysphonia and concluded that lay illness perceptions often diverge from those of the clinician which, in turn, can influence treatment behaviour. They recommend that it can be useful to explore treatment beliefs with clients so that the impact of intervention can be maximized.

A few researchers have explored the illness perceptions of parents of children with autistic spectrum condition (ASC). For example, Al Anbar, Dardennes, Prado-Netto, Kaye, & Contejean (2010) explored the ways in which parents' illness perceptions influenced their choice of treatment, including 'educational' interventions (ABA, TTEACH and PECS). Parents who perceived ASC as more serious were more likely to access educative methods and those with a higher sense of personal control were less likely to use nutritional or pharmacological methods. The authors suggest that the modification of illness perceptions may be a means of promoting evidence-based interventions and enhancing clinical outcomes (Anbar et al., 2010).

It is important to consider the illness perceptions not only of clients but also their spouses and carers. An interesting study by Twiddy, House, and Jones (2012) investigated the association between distress in stroke patients and their carers and discrepancy in their illness perceptions. They found that discrepancy in various illness perceptions can result in increased distress both for stroke survivors and their carers, highlighting the importance of health professionals having an understanding of both parties' illness perceptions to support adjustment, particularly given the role of families and carers in supporting those who have had a stroke following discharge. Similarly, Richardson, Morton, and Broadbent (2015) found that the illness perceptions of people caring for clients with head and neck cancer can contribute to the client's health-related quality of life (HRQOL); when caregivers had more negative illness perceptions, HRQOL of clients tended to be lower. Both these studies highlight the potential importance of interventions which explore illness perceptions of caregivers as well as clients themselves.

Exploring and changing illness perceptions

One way of exploring illness perceptions is through the use of case history interviews. For example, 'what do you think might be causing this?' (cause); 'what do you think might be helpful?' (coherence); 'is this affecting your mood?' (emotional representations). The Illness Perceptions Questionnaire (PPQ) website (http://www.uib.no/ipq/) contains a number of versions of the IPQ in different languages and for different 'illnesses', including autism. However, in a similar way to identifying client's 'stage of change' (see Chapter 4), they can also be explored through discussions. Van Wilgen, Beetsma, Neels, Roussel, and Nijs (2014) audiotaped the assessment consultations that physiotherapists undertook with clients with chronic lower back pain and analyzed whether illness perceptions were explored. Identity, causes and consequences were likely to be asked about whereas timeline, treatment control, coherence and emotional representation were referred to less frequently.

There is some evidence that illness perceptions can be modified and that this leads to better outcomes. For example, Broadbent, Ellis, Thomas, Gamble, and Petrie (2009) reported on an intervention aimed at modifying the illness perceptions of myocardial infarct (MI) patients. Intervention included exploration of the patient's ideas about the cause of MI, expanding these and relating them both to health behaviour and a recovery plan. Spouses were included where possible. Participants who received the intervention reported a better understanding of the information that had been given to them in hospital, higher intention to attend rehabilitation classes, less anxiety about returning to work, more increases in exercise and fewer calls to their GP (Broadbent et al., 2009, p.17). Heyduck, Meffert, and Glattacker (2014) evaluated an intervention for patients with chronic back pain that was based on the CSM.

> **Box 4.1** Illness perceptions
>
> Jane has brought her son, Ryan, aged 3 years and 3 months, to the speech and language therapist after nursery has suggested a referral. His speech is quite unintelligible, even to those who know him well. After assessment at the initial appointment, the therapist explains that Ryan has quite a significant delay in his speech sound development. She tells Jane that they will be working on /k/, which Ryan is currently realizing as /t/. In the next session, the SLT uses games in which Ryan needs to discriminate /t/ and /k/. She models the activities and asks Mum to do them at home. Mum doesn't do them and doesn't return the following week.
>
> Thinking about illness perception, why might Jane decide not to bring Ryan back to speech and language therapy? How could the therapist explore Jane's beliefs about Ryan's speech, change her illness perceptions and increase coherence?

The intervention was aimed at improving the information given to patients by incorporating an understanding of their beliefs about illness and treatment, gathered using a feedback form as a starting point. Compared with standard treatment (non-tailored information), participants in the intervention group assessed their back pain as more personally controllable and their information needs about illness and rehabilitation as having been met to a greater extent.

Stress

Stress is seemingly an unavoidable fact of life and something that professionals and clients alike will experience. As speech and language therapists, we will inevitably be exposed to various sources of stress during the course of our working lives. These might include working with clients who are very ill, distressed or 'difficult' clients and relatives, conflicts within teams, workload pressures and dealing with changing working practices. Of our clients, many are facing illness or uncertainty, dealing with bad news or coping with chronic difficulties. Attending appointments and interacting with (sometimes numerous) health, social or educational professionals can be a source of stress in itself.

The nature of stress

In the health psychology literature, stress is often considered from perspectives that concern the relationship between stress and health. A great deal of research has investigated the idea that stress *causes* illness and there seems to be evidence that this is the case (Ogden, 2012). The process by which this occurs may be via a combination of behavioural and physiological processes (Johnston, 1989). For example, individuals may attempt to control stress though engaging with unhealthy behaviours such as smoking or drinking alcohol. In addition, changes in stress-related hormones can lead to physiological changes such as raised blood pressure and decreased immune function (Ogden, 2012). There is evidence to suggest that a range of factors can mitigate against the stress–illness causal link, including coping strategies, social support and control. Our main focus in this chapter, however, is on how individuals cope with illness, disability, and the stress that can be related to these rather than the idea of stress as a *cause* of ill health.

Stressors may be major life events such as illness, bereavement and divorce that require significant adjustment on the part of the individual experiencing them. This idea stems largely from the work of Holmes and Rahe (1967) who first proposed that adjustment to major life changes increases susceptibility to physical illness. In contrast, 'daily hassles' do not require major adjustment but can nevertheless have a significant effect on wellbeing because the impact of these everyday transactions with the environment can have a cumulative effect of draining coping resources. Well-known sayings such as "any fool can face a crisis, it's the day-to-day living that wears you out" and "the straw that broke the camel's back" reflect this idea. It has been shown that this type of stress may be attenuated by 'uplifts' – small positive events such as getting enough sleep or finishing a task (Kanner, Coyne, Schaefer, & Lazarus, 1981, cited in Ogden, 2012). Many of the clients and carers with whom we work as speech and language therapists will face the major stressor of a life-changing health event or diagnosis for themselves or a loved one. Certainly, all of our clients will face 'daily hassles', be they related to their communication or swallowing difficulty (finding a car parking space for a hospital appointment; fitting in speech 'homework' with their child) or just part of the usual events that we all experience (being stuck in traffic; the dog running off). The communication or swallowing difficulty itself can also be construed as a stressor. Not only do we have a role in supporting clients to cope with stress that is directly and indirectly associated with the 'reason' we are seeing the client, we also need to be empathetic to the fact that clients have complex lives beyond the immediate speech and language concerns which have brought them to us, and that our own demands on their resources can, inadvertently, act as an additional stressor in and of themselves.

Coping with stress

Stress is often conceptualized as a transaction. The most well-known elucidation of this idea stems from the work of Lazarus and colleagues who proposed a cognitive transactional model (Lazarus & Folkman, 1984). The model considers interactions between individual characteristics such as motivational and cognitive variables; an internal or external event (the stressor itself, for example, becoming ill or a child receiving a diagnosis of autism) and the internal and external resources available to the individual to deal with the situation. There is a key role for appraisal. Primary appraisal occurs as the individual assesses the stressor, for example in terms of damage already done (harm) or expectation of future harm (threat). The stressor may also be seen as a challenge where there is an opportunity for personal growth, as might happen in a situation that a person is fairly confident they can deal with. Whilst primary appraisal is related to the potential stressor itself, secondary appraisal concerns the individual's assessment of their internal and external coping resources – in other words, their coping potential. The key idea in this model is that stress occurs when there is a mismatch between perceived demands and resources. That is, the individual does not have sufficient coping potential. It can be seen that this idea of stress as a transaction has much in common with the lifespan model of developmental challenge discussed in Chapter 3. This model, whilst being much broader in context, nevertheless describes 'resources' and 'challenges'; *development* is achieved through the successful navigation of challenging tasks. The absence of challenges may result in *stagnation*. On the other hand, if tasks are overwhelming or too 'risky' for the resources available, they may be depleted and *decay* occurs.

Strategies for coping

Coping is essentially *anything* that a person does to reduce the impact of a perceived or actual stressor. It is a dynamic process, which may be directed towards reducing negative emotions associated with the stressor or towards reducing or eliminating the stressor itself. There is an accumulating literature to suggest that supporting individuals with chronic conditions to develop a strong repertoire of coping skills is an important but sometimes neglected element of intervention by health professionals. Coping *styles* refers to a general tendency to respond to events in a particular way. They may be characterized as 'approaching', that is, paying attention to the stressor and making active efforts to deal with it versus 'avoidant' coping that is aimed at minimizing the threat. It is sometimes assumed that an approaching coping style is more adaptive but this is not always the case; distracting oneself can be an excellent coping strategy in some stressful situations, particularly those that are relatively short-term – a visit to the dentist, for example. In addition to general coping styles, individuals also use different, context-specific coping strategies. Problem-focused coping involves instrumental coping efforts aimed at either reducing demands or increasing resources. For example, the parent of a child newly diagnosed with autistic spectrum condition (ASC) may seek out information about educational options. Emotion-focused coping efforts, on the other hand, are aimed at managing the emotional response to the stressor. These might involve reappraisal of the stressor to see it in a more positive light (benefit-finding, for example) or seeking emotional support, such as talking to a friend. Attending groups may be helpful in supporting both problem-focused and emotion-focused coping; the client can get advice and ideas from others who have had similar experiences as well as having the opportunity to discuss feelings. One coping strategy is not necessarily 'better' than the other but it will depend upon a number of factors including the degree to which the stressor can be controlled. Controllability refers to the extent to which it is possible to determine or influence the desired outcome of an event or situation. Emotion-focused coping can be adaptive in uncontrollable situations, for example, a life-limiting illness such as motor neurone disease. However, setting small, achievable goals (e.g., making a 'phone call) can promote controllability.

Not all coping strategies are helpful. (Crichton-Smith, 2002) interviewed adults who stammer and found that many used social avoidance as a way of

---

Box 4.2 Reflection of a stressful situation

Think about a recent situation that you have found stressful. How did you cope with it? What different strategies did you use? Which worked and which did not? You may find it useful to try Brief COPE (Carver, 1997) to identify your preferred coping style. It is freely available at: http://www.psy.miami.edu/faculty/ccarver/sclBrCOPE.html

coping, affecting their ability to make friends and form relationships. A little later in the chapter, we look at how some ideas from positive psychology can be incorporated into practice in order to enhance coping resources.

Coping after stroke

A number of studies have explicitly explored the coping strategies of people who have experienced sudden onset illnesses such as stroke. For example, Price, Kinghorn, Patrick, and Cardell (2012) discussed the experience of a successful academic who had a stroke at a relatively young age. Social support, spirituality, internal locus of control, building on past successes (which can also be thought of in terms of 'mastery', in relation to self-efficacy, discussed further in Chapter 5), commitment to succeed, action-oriented approach and

---

Box 4.3 Coping strategies

John is a 19-year-old university student who stammers. As part of his course, he is required to give an oral presentation to a group of his peers and a tutor. Speaking in front of an audience is something that John has avoided as much as possible all his life and the prospect of it is causing him to feel stressed even through the presentation is 12 weeks away. John decides to see a speech and language therapist, something he hasn't done since he was 14.

> A long-term plan would be for John to feel comfortable to tackle this situation. However, in the short term, the therapist problem-solves with John ways in which the demands of the situation could be decreased. John agrees with his tutor that he will present in front of her and not his peers on this occasion and that he will have additional time for the presentation. These measures and fact that the tutor is now aware that John stammers have reduced the demands of the situation. John and the therapist also work on building coping resources. John plans and practises the presentation with less feared audiences, including a couple of good friends and the speech and language therapist, and this enables him to experience success, increase self-efficacy and promotes a progressive trajectory of increased coping resources. He also plans with the SLT what he will do if he experiences a severe block during the presentation. In addition to these problem-focused coping efforts, the therapist supports emotion-focused coping by working with John to identify thoughts and feelings that he has about the presentation and about stammering more generally. She also encourages him to talk with friends and family.

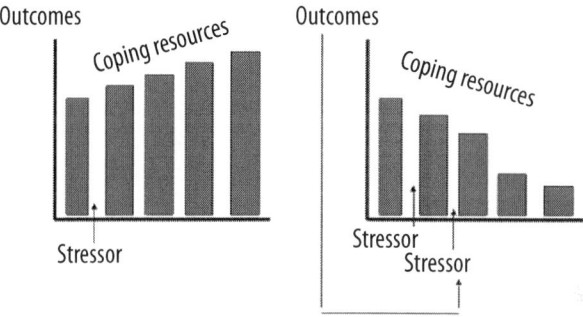

Figure 4.1 Progressive and regressive trajectories of coping after stroke
based on Kendall et al, 2007. .

having personal goals were all identified as helpful coping strategies. Williams
and Murray (2013) explored older adults' occupational adaptation following
stroke and identified 14 different coping strategies, many of which echo those
in Price. Some of these were deemed to be adaptive, including active coping
(which was associated with increased self-efficacy), emotional support, religion,
acceptance, planning, instrumental support and humour. Other strategies were
considered maladaptive and appeared be related to depression. These included
self-distraction, self-blame, denial, venting, behavioural disengagement and
substance use.

   Kendall et al. (2007) provide a useful discussion of the application of
Lazarus and Folkman's transactional theory of stress and coping to recovery
following stroke. They argue that early intervention for the psychological and
social consequences of stroke are an important but often neglected aspect of
rehabilitation that tends to focus on biomedical characteristics. They also
highlight the recursive nature of coping and adjustment; adequate coping
resources lead to better outcomes, which in turn increase coping resources.
By the same token, inadequate coping results in poorer outcomes, which then
become stressors in themselves (see Figure 4.1). The implications of this are
that early intervention is important to prevent a 'regressive trajectory' and that
the development of coping resources can promote a 'progressive trajectory'
(Kendall et al., 2007, p.737).

Aphasia following stroke is associated with stress (Hilari et al., 2010). DuBay et al. (2011) compared people with aphasia, right hemisphere brain damage and neurologically intact people. All the participants identified similar coping resources in terms of financial freedom and social support. However, people with aphasia had lower resources of stress monitoring, tension control and acceptance. Interestingly, however, although acceptance is generally considered to be a useful coping strategy, it has been found that 'insistence on recovery' (i.e., not accepting one's situation), a common characteristic of people with aphasia, is actually positively associated with functional recovery and negatively associated with depressive symptoms and apathy (DuBay et al., 2011). It is not known precisely why this is the case although the authors hypothesize that it may be because it increases motivation and allows people with aphasia to remain positive and optimistic about the future. This poses interesting questions for the speech and language therapist who may frequently find him- or herself in the position of trying to shift the focus of the client away from this idea that they will be able to recover their old communication abilities and towards encouraging the use of functional communication strategies.

Coping with a child with a disability

Research has identified that the parents of children with developmental disabilities report greater levels of stress than the parents of typically developing children (e.g., Lopes, Clifford, Minnes, & Ouellette-Kuntz, 2008). Stress can result from realizing that 'something is wrong' and receiving the diagnosis, accessing services, coping with behavioural challenges and school transitions (Lopes et al., 2008; Villeneuve et al., 2013, Brown et al., 2011, cited in Minnes, Perry, & Weiss, 2015). Positive reframing and parent empowerment have been identified as coping strategies associated with perception of positive gain for parents of children with developmental disabilities (Minnes et al., 2015).

Lai, Goh, Oei, and Sung (2015) explored the relationship between coping and wellbeing in parents of children with autistic spectrum condition. Compared to parents of typically developing children, these parents had more parenting stress symptoms and tended to use more active avoidance coping strategies. They suggest that these findings might be viewed in a cultural context; the study took place in Singapore where parents value high-achieving students and may avoid seeking help for fear of social stigma as a means of saving face (Lai et al., 2015, p.2591). Glidden and Natcher (2009) describe challenges that caregivers of children with learning disabilities may face over many years, from coping with disappointments associated with diagnosis, negotiating the health and educations systems to concerns about the future as the child grows to adulthood. They found that personality variables, particularly neuroticism, were a significant predictor of outcomes such as depression and subjective wellbeing for mothers whereas coping strategy was likely to be more important for fathers. These studies highlight the importance of the speech and language therapist remaining mindful of the way in which cultural, social as well as individual differences can impact upon preferred coping strategies and of being sensitive to these.

Health professionals: Stress, emotional labour and self-care

So far in this chapter, the focus has been on the role of stress, coping and resilience for our clients. As health professionals (and health professional students), at some time or another we are all likely to experience stress which is related to our working lives. At the severe end of the spectrum is the concept of 'burnout', defined as "a psychological syndrome in response to chronic interpersonal stressors on the job" (Maslach, Schaufell, & Lelter, 2001, cited in McManus, 2007, p.501).

Sources of occupational stress are wide ranging and might include changes in working practices, working in cramped or dilapidated buildings, feeling overloaded with work or undervalued by an employer. However, McManus (2007) points out that there is actually a rather poor correlation between variables that relate to working conditions and stress. McManus explains that the reason for this may be that, rather than workload *per se*, it is the *imbalance* of effort and reward that is problematic; a high workload may be less likely to lead to stress if the rewards are also high. An alternative explanation is that stress is related to personality variables, for example, neuroticism, of the individual professional rather than the working environment since health professionals tend to report 'poor working conditions' whether or not they report that they are stressed (McManus, 2007).

In Chapters 2 and 6 of this book, the value of emotional engagement with our clients and their families is emphasized. The ability to notice and understand emotion (what can be thought of as empathy) is a core skill for health professionals (e.g., Freshwater, 2004) and is valued by clients (e.g., Fourie, 2009). However, when we are working with clients who are experiencing suffering and grief, the quality of empathy and high levels of sensitivity to the needs of others can present challenges if we ourselves are not adequately prepared (Timmins, Corroon, Byrne, & Mooney, 2011). Indeed, Eysenck and Eysenck (1985) suggested that one's own feelings of anxiety or fear, as might be found in individuals high on neuroticism, support the ability to understand the emotional state of others. In other words, the very qualities that enable the valued characteristic of being empathetic may also result in vulnerability to stress. Anecdotally, this resonates with the authors of this book whose work with speech and language therapy students over many years has led to a recognition that many of those attracted to the profession experience heightened levels of stress throughout their studies. More broadly, as McManus points out, going home and 'worrying' about a patient, in other words, being reflective about one's practice, might very well be a desirable characteristic. Certainly, reflection is something that is widely encouraged and, indeed, required in speech and language therapy programmes and practice. For this reason, McManus counsels against any idea of selecting students on the basis of 'hardiness', since this would risk excluding the very individuals whose qualities make them sensitive and thoughtful practitioners. The implication, however, is that there needs to be appropriate support for health professionals throughout their educational and working lives.

Emotional labour

The concept of 'emotional labour' was first discussed by Hochschild in 1983 and refers to the energy that workers expend in changing or suppressing their emotions in order to comply with the expectations and 'display rules' of organizations, usually to present others (customers) with a sense of being cared for. The example discussed by Hochschild and cited by many others, refers to airline stewards who are expected to smile and display sympathy to customers whose baggage is lost where they may, in fact, feel ambivalent. These original discussions of emotional labour mainly related to commercial enterprises and the socio-political idea that emotions were being 'commodified' by large organizations. In these, as well as in some of the literature relating to health professions, the emphasis was on the requirement to express or display emotions which may not be felt. This requirement may come from the employing organization or the expectations of the profession or colleagues dictated by social and cultural norms (Badolamenti, Sili, Caruso, & Fida, 2017). A study of nurses suggested that this type of emotional labour may be used when working with patients who were perceived to be responsible for their illness or who failed to change their behaviour. In these situations, the professional context requires that healthcare professionals demonstrate empathy when this might not be felt. According to Hochschild, this outward demonstration of the required emotion may be achieved by 'surface' or 'deep' acting, that is, by 'faking' the emotional display or by attempting to put oneself in the shoes of the client so that genuine empathy – to match the demonstrated empathy – is experienced. For example, a speech and language therapist might feel anger towards the parent of a child who has missed a number of appointments and fails to follow advice yet communicates sympathy with the parent's busy life, a more socially acceptable and expected emotional offering (surface acting). On the other hand, the SLT may have developed an understanding of the challenges experienced by the client and feel genuine empathy for the parent (deep acting).

Emotional labour has been discussed somewhat more broadly in other health literature, to include 'intrapersonal' emotional labour, that is, the work involved in managing one's own emotions and those of others (Riley & Weiss, 2016). Individuals in the helping professions tend to have a high level of demand for managing emotions in terms of frequency, intensity and duration (Badolamenti et al., 2017). However, there has been some criticism of the application of the term 'emotional labour' in a healthcare context. For example, Bolton (2000) has argued that the emotion of healthcare professionals is not in fact largely commodified by organizations but that "health professionals… have the opportunity to present their 'authentic selves' in 'unmanaged spaces', places deemed free from management control" (Bolton, p.200, cited in Riley & Weiss, 2016). Job satisfaction can thus be derived from performing emotional labour and is also valued by patients (Bolton, 2000, cited in Weaver & Allen, 2017). Indeed, counselling and related contexts such as speech and language therapy place high value on the core condition of congruence, allowing clients to experience the therapist as he/she really is. Whilst arguably emotions are *not* commodified in healthcare settings, the concept of emotional labour can nevertheless provide a useful lens through which to view the management of emotions in the healthcare professions, since it is a term that seems to implicitly recognize both the *effort* required to manage emotions (be that to express a different emotion to one not felt or when no emotion is felt, or to manage one's own emotional response to dealing with clients who may be upset, angry, etc.) and the *value* that this brings to relationships and hence outcomes.

Work factors such as interpersonal conflict may also require emotional labour, for example, having a line manager who is unsupportive or having to work in a way that conflicts with one's own personal values or ideologies (Weaver & Allen, 2017). Employees who feel supported by their supervisor and able to be authentic in the company of their colleagues tend to use less emotional labour (Grandey, Foo, Groth, & Goodwin, 2012, cited in Weaver & Allen, 2017). Speech and language therapists may have a number of 'customers' or stakeholders with whom they need to manage relationships. For example, the SLT working in a school setting in a 'traded services' model needs to maintain relationships with the pupils, parents, teachers and a range of individuals who expect a good and supportive service. For speech and language therapists employed in the NHS or education sectors, the display rules may not be explicit and organizationally-imposed but they may be implicitly defined by what is appropriate and professional.

Emotion 'work' may also be undertaken away from the workplace and involve others. Those in the helping professionals may cope in the workface through using strategies such as repression but the emotions are expressed elsewhere (off-stage), for example at home, and with the support of others such as friends or family members (James, 1989, cited in Williams, 2013). Many readers will have had the experience of a 'bad day at work' resulting in fractious relations with an unsuspecting family in the evening.

Not surprisingly, workers who use higher levels of surface acting to express emotions they do not feel or to suppress emotions that they do (i.e., where there is incongruence between what is felt and what is demonstrated) tend to experience lower levels of job satisfaction and higher levels of burnout (Grandey, 2000). Burnout is associated with emotional exhaustion, depersonalisation and a reduced sense of personal accomplishment (Maslach & Jackson, 1996). It is suggested that emotional intelligence, a multidimensional concept that includes the ability to understand and regulate one's own emotions (Mayer & Salovey, 1997), makes emotional labour easier to perform and moderates the supposed negative effects of 'surface acting' such as stress, burnout and low job satisfaction (Botheridge & Grandey, 2002).

The role of emotional intelligence in stress and wellbeing of health professional students (as indicated by measures of life satisfaction and happiness) was explored in an interesting study by Ruiz-Aranda and colleagues (2014). They found that higher levels of emotional intelligence were linked to higher life satisfaction and happiness and that this link seemed to be mediated by lower levels of perceived stress. Por (2005) reported that inadequate emotional preparation was ranked as the highest stressor associated with clinical practice among healthcare students. Ruiz-Aranda et al. (2014) conclude that pre-registration health professional courses should consider building specific emotional intelligence training into the curriculum.

Support for healthcare professionals

Many authors writing about emotional labour, particularly in the healthcare professions, have identified a need for explicit training and support in contrast to the current state of affairs which tends to take the performance of emotional labour for granted. Whilst it may be a 'life skill', it is likely to be overlooked and undervalued. Many pre-registration programmes include coping skills, resilience and self-care in order to better equip students with strategies that can help them in their working lives but few, if any, explicitly refer to emotional labour or ideas associated with it. Weaver and Allen (2017) advocate explicit education in the effects of surface acting.

Many students and therapists use informal approaches to coping and managing their emotional responses to the working environment. Williams (2013) examined the strategies used by paramedic students to manage their emotional work. Strategies included informal coping mechanisms such as talking with colleagues and peers, family and friends. Students talked through experiences with their mentors and used reflection although this was sometimes seen as focusing on the technical rather than emotional aspects of practice. Interviewees also referred to the use of humour. Some speech and language therapists may find that changes in working practices, such as the use of mobile working, may mean that there are fewer informal opportunities to ameliorate the effects of emotional labour through, for example, lunchtime discussions with colleagues.

Sawbridge and Hewison (2013) note recent high profile 'failure to care' events, such as those described in *The Francis Report* and cite emotional exhaustion as one of the root causes. Again, the authors identify that changed

---

Box 4.4 Emotional labour

Thinking back to an average day of your working or placement experience, do you think that you performed 'emotional labour'? Were you hiding emotions that you did feel or expressing emotions that you didn't? What professional or social norms led you to do this? What was the impact and did you do anything specific to manage the impact?

working practices can make emotional labour more difficult to manage. The authors point to some initiatives that might help, including multidisciplinary discussion about the impact of a case on a team, clinical supervision and the approach devised by Samaritans in which buddying and debriefing are used. Other workplace strategies may include: relaxation; physical fitness; cognitive restructuring (identifying and disputing maladaptive thoughts, a key technique in cognitive behavioural therapy); assertiveness training; and stress inoculation (preparing in advance for stressful situations) (Bellarosa & Chen, 1997, cited in McManus, 2007). Manocchi (2017) discusses high levels of stress and anxiety leading to high drop-out rates among nursing students, and suggests that Mindfulness Based Stress Reduction could usefully be integrated into academic nurse education to support students in reducing stress levels, and hence increase the likelihood of using problem focused coping which, in turn, is more likely to lead to academic and clinical success. However, as yet, there is limited evidence for the effectiveness of any particular approach.

Positive psychology

So far in this chapter, the focus has primarily been on the potentially negative psychosocial impact of challenging experiences on both clients and professionals. We have also touched upon the strategies that people use to cope. Perhaps one of the most interesting developments in psychology over the past couple of decades has been that of **positive psychology**, an umbrella term for the study of positive emotions and character traits, and building an understanding of how human beings thrive and flourish (Seligman & Csikszentmihalyi, 2000). Peterson (2006) described positive psychology succinctly as "the scientific study of what goes right in life". In Holland and Nelson's (2014) excellent book focusing on a 'wellbeing perspective' of counselling in communication disorders, the authors note that the ideas of positive psychology chime well with a move away from a biomedical, disease model of health towards a biopsychosocial model of wellbeing. Ideas in positive psychology have their origin in the work of Carl Rogers and Abraham Maslow (Seligman & Csikszentmihalyi, 2000). Similar to Maslow's notion of 'self-actualization', a key concept in positive psychology is that of 'flourishing', which Seligman (2012) conceptualized in the PERMA model, containing five domains: positive emotions (P); engagement (E); relationships (R); meaning (M); and accomplishment (A). Some organizations, particularly schools, have incorporated PERMA and other positive psychology ideas into a whole approach and ethos. In January

2017, the University of Buckinghamshire announced plans to become Europe's first 'Positive University', working with Martin Seligman. Amongst a range of actions, it is proposed that every student will have a module in positive psychology, focusing on PERMA.

Character strengths are another key idea in positive psychology. Seligman and colleagues developed a classification of 24 character strengths such as curiosity, fairness, and gratitude, broadly grouped into six virtue categories: wisdom, courage, humanity, justice, temperance and transcendence (Peterson & Seligman, 2004). Online questionnaires that enable individuals to identify their 'preferred' character strengths (along with many other questionnaires and resources) are available via the Authentic Happiness website, hosted at the University of Pennsylvania (https://www.authentichappiness.sas.upenn.edu/home).

Broaden and build

Fredrickson developed the 'broaden and build' theory of positive emotions (Fredrickson, 2001). She argues that positive emotions enhance creativity and problem solving in contrast to negative emotions such as 'fight or flight' which, whilst valuable for survival, ultimately narrow one's repertoire of useful responses. Fredrickson showed that interventions, such as watching a film designed to induce happiness and positive emotion, not only increase or 'broaden' individuals' psychological, intellectual, physical and social coping resources but these outlast the positive emotions by which they were acquired and 'build' over time, increasing the individual's overall wellbeing which, in turn, leads to further positive emotions and, ultimately, lead to greater resilience (Fredrickson & Losada, 2005). What this suggests to us as speech and language therapists is that, whilst setting and supporting the achievement of goals is important, the role of boosting positive emotions, through a simple activity such as using humour or paying a compliment, should not be overlooked.

Positive psychology in therapy and rehabilitation

Positive psychology, with its focus on identification of strengths, has been influential in counselling psychology and also the 'self-help' movement, as well as the interest in embedding some of the concepts and practices into schools and other organizations. Work has been extended to 'Positive Health' which aims to research strengths that contribute to good health and protect against illness (http://positivehealthresearch.org/).

Recently, there has been interest in applying the ideas of positive psychology – and related concepts such as optimism, hope and resilience – to working with clients in rehabilitation settings as well as with people with communication difficulties. Holland and Nelson, in summarizing tenets of positive psychology, describe it as being *"as concerned with discovering strengths as it is with modulating weakness"* (p.31) and focusing *"equally on building the best things in life and repairing the worst"* (p.32), ideas which will resonate clearly with many speech and language therapists. Zebrowski and Arenas (2011) discuss strength-based intervention and positive psychology as ways of identifying and focusing on what is 'right' when working with young people who stammer and conceive this as a 'common factor' in therapy (see Chapter 2). Sharp (2012) contributed a discussion paper on the application of positive psychology in speech and language therapy. He refers to the 'primacy of positivity', suggesting that increasing the focus on clients' wellbeing and helping them to feel more positive can enhance the effectiveness of treatment. In addition to identifying and using signature strengths, Sharp (2012, p.212) suggests that it can be implemented in a number of ways including:

- Helping clients focus on and savour positive life experiences
- Finding a common interest with clients to enhance the therapeutic relationship
- Being humorous and having fun during therapy
- Cultivating a sense of hope and optimism by reminding the client of achievements
- Using evidence-based mindfulness and meditation.

Sharp also discusses the idea of 'the tyranny of when' which occurs when the client identifies a time or condition in the future when they believe they will be happy, for example, when they achieve a desirable goal such as regaining their ability to talk in the way that they used to. When the client is focused on these goals as a 'precondition' of happiness, they may ignore small pleasures in the present that can provide meaning and happiness. In addition, not only should positive emotions not be reserved until after a goal has been achieved, they should actually be viewed as a tool in and of themselves to use in the present that can lead to greater performance, coping and resilience. As in Fredrickson's 'broaden and build' theory, positive emotions broaden individuals' repertoire of coping and enables them to build on their past successes. In this way, the client may be more likely to follow a 'progressive trajectory', as outlined by Kendall et al. (2007).

Hope

In their paper on the role of hope in working with people with aphasia, Bright, Kayes, McCann, and McPherson (2013) identified three ways in which hope has been conceptualized. In a broad sense, hope can be viewed as a general state of being positive about the future. Some literature refers to this as 'generalized hope'. A second conceptualization is that of goal-oriented hope, sometimes also called particularized hope, relating to the achievement of particular goals such as eating a meal with friends or talking to a relative on the telephone. Finally, hope is seen as an active process whereby an individual is engaged in acting on hope.

In Chapter 2, expectancy was identified as an important element of the common factors model. It has been argued that the somewhat related construct of hope is important in rehabilitation and also when living with illness or injury. For example, Gum, Snyder, and Duncan (2006) found that stroke survivors with low hope tended to experience more depressive symptoms. An interesting and initially surprising finding of this study was that hopeful thinking was negatively associated with participation for participants who had poorer communication abilities. One possible reason might be that these individuals may be focused on pursuing unrealistic goals such as being able to speak in the way that they used to rather than using functional strategies such as circumlocution or a communication passport which might be more likely to improve participation. For example, using a communication passport may be associated with hopelessness because it implies that there is no possibility of change. However, it is important for the client to understand that the purpose of the passport is to enable some independent communication which itself can be a gateway to further rehabilitation. Here it is the ability to cope rather than the restoration of function that is emphasized (Soundy et al., 2014). The ability to support hope in our clients may, then, be able to contribute to positive outcomes for them. Bright et al. (2013), in their study of people with aphasia, advocated that therapists should be aware of the way in which clients experience hope, discuss hope with them clients and also engage in active intervention to support hope by, for example, providing information to reduce uncertainty and incorporating hope-supporting influences in intervention.

Teaching hope

Key ideas in hope theory (Snyder, 2002; Snyder et al., 2006) are agency (goal-directed energy) and pathways (planning to meet goals). Snyder argues that, contrary to what might be expected, it is possible to teach hope to clients. Some of the strategies for doing this are likely to be familiar to most speech and language therapists. The SLT should facilitate selection of a goal that is clearly defined and of value to the client. Importantly, the challenge level should be appropriate; goals that are too easily achieved are not effective at building agency and self-efficacy. Sub-goals should be identified and a context provided for success. Goal setting is familiar to most speech and language therapists but what they may not always pay sufficient attention to is ways they can support pathways to reaching goals. Snyder advocates the use of visualisation and generation of several paths to facilitate alternative routes. Agency can be supported through positive self-talk, by evaluating progress and increasing self-efficacy – a theme that has emerged a number of times in the course of this book. As with any change, it is important to 'mind the basics', ensuring that the client is rested, not too ill, and so on.

Optimism

Dispositional optimism has been seen as a personality variable that relates to global expectations about the future (e.g., 'everything's bound to work out') or beliefs in the face of difficulty (e.g., 'I can get through this') (Brissette, Scheier, & Carver, 2002). However, Martin Seligman and colleagues describe the idea of '*learned* optimism', contrasted with learned helplessness (M.E.P. Seligman, 2006). In response to a 'bad' event or failure, optimists tend to believe that setbacks are temporary rather than permanent, specific rather than pervasive and attributed to external causes rather than resulting from personal failure. Importantly, Seligman believes that optimism can be cultivated or learned using a version of Ellis's A (adversity) B (belief) C (consequence) rational emotive behaviour therapy (REBT) model. To this, Seligman added D (Disputations) and E (Energisation).

Adversity: I stammered when asking that girl out for a drink. She said no.

Belief: Girls think I'm stupid because I stammer and no-one will ever go out with me.

Consequence: Not asking anyone out again; becoming withdrawn.

Just as in REBT and other forms of cognitive therapy, the link between the adverse event and the consequence is challenged or disputed using techniques such as challenging the evidence (e.g., what evidence do you have that she thinks you're stupid?); drawing attention to the alternatives (e.g., are there other reasons why she might have said no?); considering implications (e.g., does this instance of a 'no' mean that every other approach will also be met with a 'no'?); and usefulness (e.g., how useful is it to you to believe that stammering makes you look stupid?). Seligman adds the idea of energisation to this process, which refers to paying attention to the way you feel as a result of disputing negative thoughts.

Optimism seems to be a predictor of successful completion of a variety of rehabilitation programmes for both children and adults (Michaels, Michaels, & Peterson, 1997). Ylvisaker and Feeney (2002) discuss the application of learned optimism in the rehabilitation of children with executive function difficulties following acquired brain injury. They note that optimism is important in initiating and maintaining goal-directed behaviour, and provide useful examples of intervention approaches which facilitate learned optimism, including the value of competent and optimistic professionals.

Resilience

Resilience refers to the ability to maintain relatively constant psychological wellbeing even in the face of loss and trauma (Bonanno, 2008). Bonanno argues that resilience is actually more common than imagined because the literature is intrinsically biased towards discussions of chronic grief and post-traumatic stress disorder. Most importantly for thinking about the relevance of resilience in working with clients, he points out that there are "multiple and sometimes unexpected paths to resilience" (Bonanno, 2008, p.107). A number of distinct dimensions are discussed including the personality traits of hardiness, self-enhancement, repressive coping and, echoing Fredrickson's broaden and build theory, positive emotion and laughter (Bonanno, 2008, pp.108-109).

White et al. (2012) used interviews to explore the trajectories of psychological distress after stroke. They identified a 'resilience' trajectory which was underpinned by adaptability (for example to different surroundings or circumstances), previous life experiences (such as poverty or being in the war), optimism, and an altered life perspective ('lucky to be alive'). However, participants with cognitive or language impairments were excluded. Fromm et al. (2011) reported a study in which they asked people with aphasia about their speech. Whilst acknowledging that participants in the sample were self-selecting, they comment on their general propensity to talk in positive terms. The authors reflect that healthy people tend to underestimate the self-reported wellbeing of people with chronic disability, and that focusing on positive experiences when faced with hardship may be an important part of the adaptation process. They cite a study by Cruice, Worrall, Hickson and Murison (2009) who found that the spouses of people with aphasia tended to rate their quality of life lower than the people with aphasia themselves (p.1143). Fromm and colleagues invite therapists to work with their clients to explore and identify their 'resilience factors' from their pre-stroke lives which may help to encourage resilient behaviours, strengthen their sense of self in the altered context of living with aphasia, and improve outcomes.

Box 4.5 Case example

John and Maggie have a daughter, Jade, who has Down Syndrome. Jade is now 7 years old and the differences between her and her peers is becoming more evident, particularly in terms of her communication. Her understanding is at an approximately 4;6 level and she is often unintelligible. This is affecting her relationships and behaviour at her mainstream school.

As a speech and language therapist, identify at least two ways in which you could use the ideas introduced in this chapter when working with Maggie, John and Jade.

Conclusions

In this chapter, a number of ideas from the health psychology and other literature that are relevant to speech and language therapy have been explored. Understanding the beliefs that our clients have about their communication or swallowing difficulties is an important though often overlooked strategy for increasing adherence; we cannot assume that clients' understanding of their difficulties is the same as our own. Although broad in scope, many overlapping themes have emerged in relation to coping and resilience. Supporting clients to develop their coping resources and discover their own paths to resilience is a critical part of our role. In Chapter 6, we consider some practical approaches to the therapeutic process which can support this. Finally, it needs to be acknowledged that, whilst there are many reasons to believe that the ideas and principles discussed here are valuable when working with clients, empirical research, particularly intervention studies, are limited to non-existent. As we outlined in Chapter 1, we hope that this situation will change over the next decade.

5 Changing behaviour

Introduction

Regardless of the field or specialist area, the work of speech and language therapists almost always involves advising people (clients, carers, parents, teachers, nurses, healthcare or teaching assistants and so on) to do something beyond the activities that take place in an actual 'therapy session'. In some cases, this may be specific and time limited, for example, the parent who is advised to do speech sound activities with their child once a day for six weeks or the teaching assistant who is asked to implement a speech and language therapy programme for a child with a language disorder over the course of a half term. This type of intervention might typically (though not always) apply to 'impairment-based' interventions, where the aim is to 'cure' or produce a measurable change in speech, language or swallowing function itself. These types of activities require that clients *adhere* to the advice or 'homework' provided by the speech and language therapist. In other cases, change of a different nature is called for. These sorts of changes require the client (or other individual) to make changes in their behaviour that are typically more pervasive in the sense that they need to become a part of everyday life (as opposed to being an 'event' which happens at a specific time of day) and are often not time limited (i.e., something to be done for six weeks, etc.). These types of intervention are usually, though not exclusively, associated with functional therapy where the aim is for adjustment to or compensation for a communication or swallowing difficulty that is unlikely to undergo major change or improvement in itself. Examples might include: vocal hygiene; using high- and low-tech AAC; using strategies to enhance intelligibility; modified diets. These types of activities emphasize the role of *self-management*, with the expectation being that the client or carer is supported to take responsibility for ongoing management of communication or swallowing needs. Indeed, a short web search suggests that many speech and language therapy services refer explicitly in their publicly-available information to the role of self-management for all types of difficulties. This trend is likely to continue in line with political, social and economic drivers such as NHS reforms, patient empowerment and an emphasis on proactive management of chronic disease (Naylor et al., 2013) as well as an era of budgetary constraint. The NHS Five Year Forward View has set out priorities for a sustainable NHS and includes specific reference to supporting people to manage their own health. For speech and language therapists and their managers, this is already translating into changes in working practices such as a 'skill mix' agenda and a prevailing climate of SLTs in some contexts using a consultative model.

Alongside and frequently overlapping with the role of self-management, there is increasing recognition of the value of a public health or *health promotion* role for speech and language therapy. A typical activity here might be providing information to parents, carers and other health workers or educators about what they can do to support children's communication development (e.g., Ferguson & Spence, 2012). Again, this trend is likely to continue in the context of prevention as a national picture in health care.

Given these aspects of speech and language therapy work, it is puzzling that relatively little attention has been paid to how we might be able to enhance the effectiveness of these types of interventions within the context of evidence-based practice. Regardless of the specific disorder or management approach, therapeutic change is unlikely where individuals do not effect actions that are recommended or, in other words, where they do not practise tasks outside the therapy environment or integrate changes to behaviour into their daily lives. It is critical for effective practice that the individuals who are largely responsible for implementing changes have the maximum chance of being able to make and maintain those changes. For this reason, theories and techniques of *behaviour change*, taken primarily from the field of health psychology, are likely to be highly relevant to speech and language therapy practice. Whilst relatively little empirical research on their application in a specific speech and language therapy context currently exists, we can nonetheless extrapolate research and ideas that have been done in other areas in order to enhance our practice.

In the rest of this chapter, we will outline some key ideas in adherence and behaviour change from the health psychology and other literature and make use of clinical examples to illustrate how they might be used to enhance speech and language therapy practice.

Adherence

Adherence has been extensively studied, particularly in the field of medicine. Almost all speech and language therapy intervention involves direct input from a therapist and advice about activities for clients or carers to carry out between sessions. Non-adherence to advice or activities is likely to have a significant impact on treatment outcome and, in some cases, may even be dangerous (non-adherence to modified diet advice, for example). In considering the relationship between behaviour change and adherence, perhaps adherence might be thought of as more relevant to activities that are of limited duration and somewhat circumscribed (for example, the parent who practises /s/ words with his child between therapy sessions) whereas behaviour change tends to be discussed in relation to more durable and pervasive actions (for example, the adult with aphasia who uses a communication book). From a practical point of view, this is probably of less importance than the ability to select and use strategies from the 'behaviour change and adherence toolbox' to improve effectiveness when working with clients. The term 'adherence' is used more commonly now than 'compliance' as it is seen as reflecting a more equal balance of power between the professional and the client.

There are many reasons why clients do not or cannot comply with healthcare instructions. Clearly, medical reasons such as acute illness can impact upon and affect the individual's capacity to adhere, and behaviours such as drug and alcohol addiction may impair the individual's capacity to self-manage their own health care. In an extensive discussion of factors affecting compliance in the rehabilitation setting Millslagle (http://www.d.umn.edu/~dmillsla/documents/PTpresentationf09.pd) discusses the practical aspects of difficulties with adherence such as access to rehabilitation and transport, the client's perception of the rehabilitation process and general psychosocial factors such as stress and anxiety. Wittig and Schurr's (1994) study also reports professionals' views on factors affecting adherence such as the client's overestimation of the effectiveness of the rehabilitation and their general hardiness and resilience in this context.

There are, however, less obvious factors that may make adherence difficult to achieve. One of the areas most studied focuses on the effect of cognition on compliance. DiMatteo and DiNicola (1982) examined doctor-patient communication in relation to compliance, and many of these results can be applied to other healthcare contexts. Firstly, they found that patients forget much of what the doctor tells them and that the more they are told, the more they will forget. Interestingly, they also found that more intelligent patients do not remember more than less intelligent patients. In relation to anxiety levels while seeing the doctor, DiMatteo and DiNicola found that those who were assessed as moderately anxious patients recalled more about what they were told than highly anxious patients, or patients who were not anxious at all.

The cognitive hypothesis model of adherence

Ley (1988) introduced the cognitive hypothesis model of adherence which predicts that patients are more likely to adhere to treatment if they understand and remember what they have been told and are satisfied with the consultation or appointment.

Memory

Ley (1997) identified that 75% of information given in four statements is likely to be retained compared with 50% in 10 statements. Strategies for enhancing memory include presenting information in a structured and organized way and repeating key information. Saliency and recency effects should be considered; clients are more likely to remember information if it seems relevant to them and are also more likely to remember the last thing that was said. Therapists should also be explicit in stressing the importance of 'doing' what they are being asked to do. Written material can be helpful but it is important to go through this with clients, highlighting the elements that are most relevant to him or her as an individual, particularly if the written material is in the form of a generic leaflet, for example, on encouraging language development or providing vocal hygiene advice; this is likely to increase the saliency of the information for clients.

Understanding

Simple strategies such as avoiding jargon and checking the client's understanding can be helpful here. It is also important to relate the 'action' required to the cause. Illness perceptions are the beliefs that people hold about their condition such as how long it will last and what caused it. These were discussed more fully in Chapter 4 but it is easy to see, for example, why the father bringing a child with unintelligible speech to therapy may not understand why activities are focused on listening rather than speaking. This may affect his adherence to listening activities that the speech and language therapist asks them to practise at home. It is worth recognizing that special attention will often be needed with speech and language therapy clients in order to support them to understand and remember information given to them.

Satisfaction

In the modern NHS, patient satisfaction is seen as a critical part of the provision of services and all providers gather feedback from clients in some form, for example, the 'family and friends test'. Satisfaction is likely to depend on the affective aspects of the appointment session, including the clinician's demonstration of emotional support and understanding. The importance of the therapeutic relationship is discussed further in Chapter 2. Some research has also shown that high satisfaction is related to the use of light humour such as humour that relieves tension or is self-effacing (Sala, 2002, in Ogden, 2012).

Perceptions and practicalities approach

An alternative model of adherence, the perceptions and practicalities approach, was proposed by Horne (2001) who made a useful distinction between unintentional and intentional non-adherence. Unintentional non-adherence generally arises as a result of capacity and resource limitations such as lack of time or failing to remember. There may be additional practical barriers; for example, the teaching assistant who is unable to find a free room to carry out the programme that the speech and language therapist has left. On the other hand, intentional non-adherence can arise because of the way that clients perceive their difficulty. For example, the parent with the language-delayed child may believe that he or she will just 'catch up' and therefore lack the motivation to do the activities suggested by the speech and language therapist.

Adherence in speech and language therapy

A few studies have explored factors that affect adherence in speech and language therapy interventions. Dysphagia is clearly an area where there may be significant consequences to not adhering to treatment advice. Reasons for non-adherence to dysphagia advice may include: denial of having a swallowing problem; dissatisfaction with thickened fluids and pureed food; minimising the severity of the problem; and taking a 'calculated risk' in deciding not to adhere to advice (Colodny, 2005). Chadwick et al. (2006) explored caregivers' barriers to following eating and drinking advice when working with clients with learning disability. Barriers included practical problems with posture and positioning, concern about the potential for conflict between what the person wants and the recommended diet, and fear of making mistakes.

Van Leer and Connor (2015) identified a number of barriers to clients' adherence to behavioural voice therapy. These included forgetting how to reproduce a target voice technique without the therapist being present, difficulty judging the accuracy of their attempts, and worries about sounding unnatural when using the target technique in conversation. Other influencing factors included self-efficacy (confidence in being able to perform a specific action, discussed later in this chapter) and therapeutic alliance (discussed in Chapter 2) and accounted for a significant amount of variance in adherence. They used a mobile video intervention consisting of peer, self and clinician modelling of techniques and found that participants who received the video intervention had greater self-efficacy for generalisation than those who had the standard voice therapy alone (van Leer & Connor, 2015). Over the coming years, the widespread availability of mobile technology, including smartphones, holds promise in supporting clients to adhere to treatment advice.

There has been some interest in the role of self-regulation (sometimes referred to as self-control) in adherence to voice therapy. Self-regulation is seen as an aspect of executive function and refers to an individual's ability to monitor and control their own behaviour, emotions or thoughts as required by the demands of a situation (Vohs & Baumeister, 2004). It is considered to be a resource that can be depleted or 'used up' when sustained over time (for example, a person may control irritation with a colleague at work during the day but snap at the family when they get home) but which can be restored with rest (i.e., in circumstances where it is not being used, such as when relaxing or experiencing positive mood). Vinney and Turkstra (2013) provide a useful summary of self-regulation in relation to adherence and changing health behaviours such as exercising and dieting and discuss its potential as an important construct in 'physiological' voice therapies such as Lee Silverman Voice Therapy (El Sharkawi et al., 2002) and accent method (Thyme & Frøkjær-Jensen, 2001). During the skills acquisition phase, these therapies typically involve learning to produce particular vocal techniques, making changes to motor behaviour via specific vocal exercises with input from the therapist. Self-regulation is required at this stage to refine the voice production in order to achieve the new target accurately. In the habit formation and habit change phase, these new voice behaviours are gradually transferred to everyday speech across different environments with fewer self-regulatory resources required over time. Vinney and Turkstra (2013) outline a number of ways in which self-regulation can 'fail' during voice therapy. For example, the client may be unable to form a mental representation or motor program for the new vocal behaviour during the skill acquisition phase, or an incompatible goal (e.g., raising the voice at a busy dinner table) may be activated at the same time as the goal of using the new behaviour during the habit formation phase (Vinney & Turkstra, 2013, p.390). They suggest that implementation intentions (discussed below) may be a way of reducing the load on cognitive resources and, hence, self-regulatory demands. Vinney, van Mersbergen, Connor, and Turkstra (2016) reported a 'proof-of-concept study' in which they further explored the role of self-regulation in voice clients. There was preliminary evidence that clients in a self-regulation depletion condition (writing about a recent vacation without using the letters 'a' or 'n') subsequently performed less well in using vocal modification during a speaking task than clients in a control group. However, a relaxation intervention, hypothesized to 'replete' self-regulation resources in this study, did not have any effect. Although in the early stages of investigation, the concept of self-regulation and self-regulation depletion may prove a useful concept for speech and language therapists to consider when working with a range of client groups. For example, the timing and structuring of practice tasks to avoid points of high self-regulatory depletion and reduce cognitive demands, e.g., through the use of implementation intentions, could be considered.

Adherence factors in written material

In addition to the interaction between healthcare professional and patient, there is also work which has examined the methods used to give patients instructions about health information. Written information can be a powerful aid to enable patients to follow their health instructions effectively. Hoffman and Worral (2004) note that using written information can provide consistency over time as the patient can refer to it when required, it can help recall, and the information is portable. Ley (1988) notes that written information should be supported by verbal information so that the patient receives the information through two mediums.

Various researchers have been interested in the complexity of written materials in relation to the individual's capacity to comply. The comprehensibility of written materials is influenced by the readability of the material and also, importantly, by the patient's reading ability. Pothier et al. (2008) examined 20 existing health information leaflets which were available in a Speech and Language Therapy Department in the UK. The leaflets were analyzed in terms of their readability and only 25% of the leaflets met standards of readability for the general population. Thus, although the health information leaflets were available to help patients, in practice they may only have been of limited use. In a useful follow-up to these findings, Pothier et al. (2008) then revised the leaflets using a NHS Toolkit for producing patient information which showed an improvement in the readability statistics in the length of components including average word counts, number of sentences and paragraphs. In addition, complexity was reduced following the improvements, ensuring that the revised leaflets were more appropriate for this population.

In order to analyze the readability of written material, various measurements have been devised. A commonly used approach is that of the SMOG rating (Simple Measure of Gobbledegook) which can be used to analyze a written piece of material. It involves counting the words of three or more syllables in 3 × 10-sentence samples, estimating the count's square root, and adding 3. This will give a reading level which can be compared to reading levels used in educational settings.

Another well-known method of testing reading levels is the Flesch–Kincaid readability tests, designed to indicate how difficult a reading passage in English is to understand. This method includes two tests, the Flesch reading ease, and the Flesch–Kincaid grade level. Although both use the same core measures (word length and sentence length), they have different weighting factors. Further guidance may be found on the Readibility Formulas website (http://www.readabilityformulas.com/flesch-grade-level-readability-formula. php) and this approach is used worldwide.

Herbert et al. (2012) undertook a study to determine what aspects of written information needed to be taken into account in order to ensure the material was accessible to people with aphasia. Some clear themes emerged from the study which asked aphasia speakers to examine different written and visual styles. There emerged five key requirements: a short message; clear sentences; easy words; good layout; and making a set. In a booklet published by the Stroke Association (stroke.org.uk), Herbert et al. describe the five themes with guidance about how to create accessible written material. Further advice about suitable approaches to word processing for this population, including the use of the Flesch–Kincaid test in Accessible Information Guidelines, is available at the Stroke Association website (https://www.stroke.org.uk/sites/ default/files/accessible_information_guidelines.pdf1_.pd).

Health behaviours and theories of behaviour change

Older definitions of 'health behaviours' have generally focused on activities that are undertaken by a person who is currently healthy in order to prevent disease or to detect disease before it becomes symptomatic (Connor & Norman, 2005). Examples might include engaging in certain 'healthy behaviours' such as eating healthily (for example, eating five portions of fruit and vegetables a day); avoiding 'unhealthy behaviours' such as smoking or excessive alcohol consumption; and attending preventative screen programmes such as cervical smear or self-examination for prostate cancer. Such a definition would undoubtedly encompass the public health or health promotion role of speech and language therapy practice. Connor and Norman (2005) make a case for extending this definition because it does not include activities undertaken by people who have a diagnosis or condition (for example, diabetes, high blood pressure) that are directed as self-management, be this to prevent worsening of the condition or to improve wellbeing whilst not eliminating the condition. They suggest that "*a useful broad definition would include any activity undertaken for the purpose of preventing or detecting disease or for improving health and well-being*" (Connor & Norman, 2005, p.2). We can certainly recognize many of the activities of speech and language therapists and their clients as being encompassed by this latter definition. Michie and Johnston (2012) have emphasized the importance of defining behaviour in behaviour change research and suggest the following definition:

> "Anything a person does in response to internal or external events. Actions may be overt (motor or verbal) and directly measurable, or covert (e.g. physiological responses) and only indirectly measurable; behaviours are physical events that occur in the body and are controlled by the brain."
> *Hobbs, Campbell, Hildon, & Michie, 2011, cited in*
> *Michie & Johnston, 2012, p.2*

Michie and Johnston (2012) point out that behaviour may refer to simple, specific actions. A speech and language therapy example might be adding thickener to a drink or undertaking a daily phonology activity with a child. More usually, however, behaviour in the context of health is more complex and involves a series of actions that take place over time. For example, in a speech and language therapy context, it might involve parents making a series of adaptations in the way they interact with their child to promote speech and language development. The influence of client behaviour is important both in preventing illness or other difficulties in the first place and in managing chronic, long-term difficulties (Hibbard & Gilburt, 2014).

There are numerous theories of behaviour change. A project led by Susan Michie and colleagues has specifically sought to build a taxonomy of theories. In total, 93 distinguishable theories were identified although, as you might expect, many overlap or contain similar constructs (Michie et al., 2013). An interesting observation from this work was that 13 theories accounted for almost 90% of articles found. Very many of the theories have potential to be valuable in speech and language therapy practice. Below, we will consider three theories and their application in practice: the Transtheoretical Model of Change, one of the best known and most widely-used theories applied to behaviour change; the Health Action Process Approach, which has its roots in social cognitive theory and emphasizes the role of self-efficacy; finally, COM-B, a relatively recent model that forms part of an extensive and detailed account of behaviour change developed by Susan Michie and colleagues and provides a framework for 'behavioural diagnosis' and intervention.

Transtheoretical Model of Change

The Transtheoretical Model of Change (TTM), sometimes known as the 'Stages of Change' model, was developed by Prochaska and DiClemente (1982) and is based on a synthesis of different psychotherapies that involved eliciting and maintaining change (Ogden, 2012). The theory is 'transtheoretical' in the sense that it is not specific to any particular therapy approach but can be applied across them. The model proposes that people gradually move through a series of identifiable stages when changing behaviour. It also recognizes that they are unlikely to move in a linear way through the stages but may 'spiral', returning to earlier stages before moving forward again. An important concept in the TTM is 'readiness': successful movement through the stages requires that individuals must be *ready* to move from one stage to the next.

Stages of change

Prochraska and Prochraska (1999) described the stages through which clients pass:

> **Precontemplation**: At this stage, individuals typically do not recognize a need for change. They may not recognize that there is a problem or, when weighing up the pros and cons, may underestimate the potential positive impact of change or overestimate the negative aspects of changing. For example, a teenager who stammers may be encouraged to attend a speech and language therapist by a parent but have little interest in engaging with a therapy process at that point.

Contemplation: According to Prochaska, clients at this stage usually intend to change within the next six months. They may be engaged in 'decisional balance'; they are weighing up the costs and benefits associated with change but are not yet ready for active behavioural change. For example, the parent of a child with language delay may be considering attending a language group but have concerns about the time commitment and be uncertain about the value of the group.

Preparation: Clients at this stage may be taking small steps towards change. They may be seeking information on the web, trying to make some changes themselves or, if they have not already done so, identifying professionals or other individuals who can help.

Action: At this stage, tangible change is happening. This may be at the level of individual behaviours – what Prochaska and DiClemente (1986) refer to as the symptom or situational level – or, more profoundly, changes related to one's thoughts and beliefs, personal relationships or sense of self. For example, a client with dysarthria may be actively using strategies to enhance intelligibility which may be indicative of change at the situational level and beyond.

Maintenance: This stage involves active attempts to prevent relapse. There is likely to be less active change than in the action stage, for example in the form of practice, but continued conscious effort is needed to achieve lasting change. For example, following discharge, an individual with expressive aphasia may choose to become involved in a support group where they can gain social support and practise total communication strategies learned in therapy.

A key clinically useful aspect of the TTM is that it explains how *different therapeutic strategies* or change processes are likely to be effective with clients who are at *different stages of change*. It is therefore important for a speech and language therapist to identify the stage that a client is 'at' and match their intervention strategies accordingly since 'strategy to stage mismatch' is likely to result in the client not progressing through the stages to succeed in making and maintaining therapeutic change.

Recognizing stages and selecting approaches

A 'Stages of Change Questionnaire' was developed by McConnaughy, Prochaska and Velicer (1983) and subsequently adapted for use with various populations, including people who stutter (Floyd, Zebrowski, & Flamme, 2007). Its main use, however, has been to provide empirical evidence for the TTM in research rather than as a clinical assessment tool. For the majority of speech and language therapists, the most practical way of identifying the stage that a client is at is likely to be through discussion and careful listening. Whilst it is probably unrealistic and unnecessary to make a fine-grained differentiation

---

Box 5.1 Stages of change

Read the following comments by clients and try to identify what stage you think they might be on the TTM, based on the descriptions above. Don't worry if you can't quite decide between a couple of stages. What change processes and interventions might be particularly helpful?

1. I was going to use the VOCA (Voice Output Communication Aid) but it wasn't charged.

This client seems to be in contemplation or preparation stage. According to the TTM, important processes here might be self-revaluation and self-liberation. The SLT might spend time exploring the client's self-concept and how using the VOCA might impact on this. Problem solving and gaining a commitment to a specific action might be helpful too; this could involve exploring barriers to charging the VOCA and agreeing a small, achievable goal with the client.

2. I noticed that when I spoke more slowly, people seemed to understand me better.

The client seems to be in action stage. Helping relationships are important here. The SLT could be providing positive feedback and reinforcement for the actions already taken and working with the client to identify further goals, encouraging him or her to try the strategy in different situations, with the SLT and client evaluating the results together.

3. I don't see why speaking more slowly is going to help – we were just the same with his brother and he doesn't stammer.

This client is probably in pre-contemplation stage. Consciousness raising and dramatic relief are particularly relevant processes here. The SLT could spend time exploring parents' feelings about stammering. It would also be important to explain the rationale for reducing speaking rate and relate this to theories about stammering. Asking parents to make changes to their speaking rate at this stage might not be effective.

Table 5.1 Stages of Change and Change Processes.

Stage of change	Recognized by	Change process	Definition (based on Michie et al., 2014, pp.448–449)	Examples from SLT
Pre-contemplation	The client is not intending to make any changes.	Consciousness raising	Provide accurate information about the issue or problem.	Providing information about speech and language development to the parent of a child with language delay.
		Dramatic relief	Expressing feelings about the problem and solution.	The therapist uses counselling skills (alongside other resources, such as a Blob Tree) to explore a teenage client's feelings about stammering and therapy.
Contemplation	Client is considering making changes. May say things such as	Environmental re-evaluation	Assessment of how a behaviour might impact on the social environment.	A client with PD considers whether strategies for intelligibility would enable him to reach a meaningful goal such as going for a drink with some friends.
		Self re-evaluation	Assessment of self-image in relation to the problem.	The SLT explores a client with Ms's feelings towards using an alternative mean of communication.
		Self-liberation	Belief in ability to change a particular behaviour and commitment to act on it.	
Preparation	Client starts making small changes	Helping relationships	Relationships that are supportive of the behaviour change.	The SLT and client agree a goal of making a telephone call. The client commits to a time and place for making the call.
Action	Client is actively engaging in a new behaviour.	Counter conditioning	Adoption of the desired behaviour as a substitute for a 'problem' behaviour.	The SLT explores with the client their current situation, the preferred situation and identifies actions to get there. Provided positive feedback for changes made.
Maintenance	The client is maintaining the new behaviour over time.	Stimulus control	Reduce cues for problem behaviour and increase cues for new behaviour.	The parent of a child with language delay commits to turning the television off for 20 minutes per day after their favourite programme has finished.
		Reinforcement management	The person is 'rewarded' by themselves or others for engaging in the desired behaviour or 'punished' for not engaging in desired behavior.	The SLT works with a voice client to identify specific situations where they might shout and identifies whether this situation could be avoided or what could be done instead. The parent of a child uses stickers as a reward after practising speech sound homework for 10 minutes each day.
		Social liberation	Noticing social, policy or environmental changes.	The client with a voice disorder notices that it is becoming almost impossible to find indoor places to smoke.

between all five stages (and, indeed the work of McCoaughy, Prochaska and Velicer (1983) implied that a separate 'preparation' stage may not be useful) it *is* important to be able to recognize that, for example, attempting to elicit 'action' in clients who are in contemplation or even pre-contemplation is likely to be unsuccessful.

Health Action Process Approach

Another example of a stage model that is frequently described in the health psychology literature is the Health Action Process Approach (HAPA) (Schwarzer, 1992; Schwarzer & Fuchs, 1995). The HAPA includes elements from social cognition models and emphasizes the role of *self-efficacy*. It explores factors that facilitate the adoption and maintenance of health behaviours in at least two stages: a motivational stage whereby an individual develops an intention, and an action phase that considers how cognitive and situational factors influence behaviour change.

Risk perception

Risk perceptions involve an individual's appraisal of threat both in terms of the seriousness of the threat and their own vulnerability to it. For example, a person with dysphagia considering a modified diet might consider whether her risk of getting pneumonia was high, average or low compared with other people in her situation. Although risk perception is included in the HAPA, it is considered as having limited value in explaining intentions compared to other factors.

Outcome expectancies

Outcome expectancies refer to the 'pros and cons' of what a person expects to happen if they undertake a change in behaviour. For example, a client given vocal hygiene advice might have a positive outcome expectancy that "if I drink more water, my voice will improve" and a negative outcome expectancy that "if I drink more water, I will have to go to the toilet every 5 minutes".

Self-efficacy

An important construct in health psychology literature is **self-efficacy**, postulated by Bandura (1977) as a unifying theory of behavioural change; it is included in many models of behaviour change and was later expanded as part of his social learning theory (Ogden, 2012). Self-efficacy is "the belief in one's capabilities to organize and execute the sources of action required to manage prospective situations" (Bandura, 1995, p.2). One way of thinking about it is as confidence related to a specific situation. Self-efficacy is thought to have an important impact on how people approach tasks and goals, and individuals with high self-efficacy for behaviour X are more likely to succeed in achieving behaviour X. A potentially useful activity for the SLT is to work with a client in developing a series of self-efficacy statements, which can then be rated by the client. This provides an opportunity to explore explicitly with clients the potential barriers to carrying out behaviours and therefore elicit helpful information that can serve to direct the focus of problem solving.

Sources of self-efficacy

Bandura (1977) discusses four important sources of self-efficacy.

Mastery: Mastery experiences are the most important source of self-efficacy. Put simply, it refers to the idea that an individual is more likely to believe that they can succeed in a task if they have previously done so. This implies that, as speech and language therapists, it is important for us to carefully select tasks and targets for our clients that will result

---

Box 5.2 Self-efficacy

Jane is a paediatric speech and language therapist working with the parents of Simon, a 3;5-year-old boy who has been stammering for about 9 months. Jane advised parents to spend 5 minutes per day in non-directive play with Simon. Jane works with Simon's Mum to identify potential challenges to her being able to implement special time and develop a series of self-efficacy statements:

- I am confident that I can do 'special time' every day even if...
  - I am feeling really tired
  - I get back late from work
  - Simon's younger brother is demanding attention

in success most of the time (since the occasional failure in the context of many successes is not seen as problematic) whilst being sufficiently challenging as to lead to meaningful gains and development.

Vicarious learning: Seeing others succeed in activities is another important source of self-efficacy. Effectiveness is likely to be increased if the behaviour is demonstrated more than once by a variety of models whose characteristics are personally relevant to the individual and if the behaviour is shown to result in positive outcomes rather than simply be 'ends in themselves' (Bandura, 1977). There are a number of implications of this. Clients' self-efficacy is likely to be enhanced if they have the opportunity to observe the behaviour being demonstrated by people in the same situation as they are rather than by the clinician alone. One obvious way to accomplish this is via a group therapy setting where individuals can observe and learn from each other. The role and value of group therapy as well as self-led support groups is discussed further in Chapter 6. In addition, being able to observe the success in a 'real life' situation with a 'real life' consequence will be more helpful than simply practising or observing in the clinic or at home. This suggests that intervention should be 'taken out of the clinic room' wherever possible. For example, visiting a café with more experienced members of a stroke group would enable a new member to observe others using Total Communication strategies to effectively order a drink. It has to be recognized, however, that resources such as time and staffing may limit the opportunity for group or 'beyond-clinic' activities. It may be necessary – and increasingly possible – to be creative in facilitating vicarious learning opportunities through, for example, telehealth and social media.

Verbal persuasion: Verbal persuasion alone is seen as a weak predictor of effective performance because it does not include any experience of success (either one's own or that of others) in and of itself. However, encouragement can be helpful in developing confidence, particularly where its source is credible, for example, the friend or relative who knows the client well or the experienced therapist who is able to draw on working with clients with similar difficulties. Constructive and accurate feedback can also help to develop self-efficacy.

Emotional arousal: As many people will be able to reflect, confidence can be significantly affected by moods, emotion and stress. General low mood or feeling highly anxious about a specific situation can have a negative impact on self-efficacy. For this reason, it is important for the speech and language therapist to be aware of what else is happening in the client's life and be realistic about how that affects clients' confidence and, ultimately, their engagement in therapy. It may also be useful to discuss specific strategies for controlling nerves relating to specific situations, for example breathing techniques.

Implementation intentions

Although the HAPA does not specifically include the concept of implementation intentions, the notion of planning is an important construct in the model. As any of us who have ever attempted to make changes to our behaviour are all too aware, it is not unusual for there to be a 'gap' between the *intention* to carry out a particular behaviour and the *reality* of actually doing it. Gollwitzer (1999) introduced the idea of *implementation intentions* to explain how the intention "I intend to do more exercise" is more likely be translated into "I have begun to exercise" if the individual has a simple but detailed plan of when, where and how the behaviour is going to happen (for example, "I will go for a walk tomorrow lunchtime after I have finished teaching"). Numerous studies have supported the effectiveness of implementation intentions. For

---

Box 5.3 Implementation intentions

Helen is aged 9 years. She has cerebral palsy and learning disability.

- Goal: Use VOCA during day trip with family.
- Sub-goals (for Mum): (1) Identify appropriate vocabulary. (2) Ensure vocab available on VOCA. (3) Practise vocab in structured situation.
- Plan (for sub-goal 3): When – Thursday evening after 'Hollyoaks'; where – in the kitchen (no TV); and how – with Mum, Dad, younger brother using cue-cards in board game.
- Feedback: Ask Mum to note any difficulties (at the time, e.g., using structured form); discuss with therapist; problem solve; form new plan as needed.
- Support: School involvement (e.g., contact TA); identify training for VOCA programming.

example, Sheeran and Orbell (2000) found that women who were due for a cervical smear test were asked to write down **when**, **where**, and **how** they would make an appointment. These women were more likely to actually attend for screening compared with controls who were equally motivated to attend but did not specify their implementation intention. The simple notion guides us to be specific with our clients by introducing a situational cue to a specific behaviour; rather than "please practise before I see you next week", work with the client to identify *when, where* and *how* they will practise.

Bandura (2000) identified that successful change depends upon identifying agreed goals and a set of achievable sub-goals, devising a plan of action (specifying) where, when and how, providing feedback on performance and the availability of support.

Contemporary approaches to behaviour change: The Behaviour Change Wheel, COM-B, and behaviour change taxonomy

The Behaviour Change Wheel, COM-B

COM-B is a relatively new model of behaviour change and forms part of a very comprehensive body of work undertaken by Susan Michie and colleagues in which a step-by-step process for designing behaviour change interventions is described. The steps are discussed in detail in a book, *The Behaviour Change Wheel* (BCW; Michie, Atkins, & West, 2014) which also provides worked examples and worksheets enabling readers to undertake the process in their own settings. The steps described in the BCW include specifying precisely what behaviours need to change in order to bring about a desired outcome and prioritizing and selecting a target behaviour based on criteria such as evidence for its likely impact. For example, safe management of clients with swallowing problems requires a number of behaviours such as using the correct amount of thickener in drinks, blending food to the right consistency, correct use of specialist equipment such as spoons and cups, ensuring residents are positioned correctly, helping clients to eat, observing clients for signs of aspiration. Of these, the SLT might decide to prioritize 'using the correct amount of thickener' and this specific target behaviour needs to be described in detail, for example, who performs it, when and where.

A core element of the process described in the BCW is identifying precisely *what* needs to change by performing a behavioural diagnosis using the COM-B.

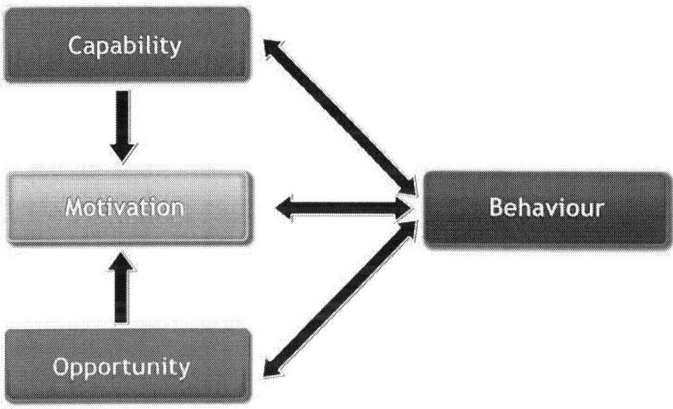

Figure 5.1 COM-B. Reproduced by permission of Silverback Publishing (part of Silverback Internet Services Limited) from the publication *The Behaviour Change Wheel.*

According to the COM-B system, a behaviour at any particular moment occurs as a result of an individual's capability, motivation and opportunity to perform it. (Michie et al., 2014). COM-B therefore provides a framework of interacting elements for identifying *precisely* what needs to change in order for a target behaviour to occur. (As an aside, many readers may notice how the ideas in the COM-B seem to have many similarities to Della Money's 'means, reasons and opportunities' model; that is, 'capability' is equivalent to 'means' and 'motivation' is equivalent to 'reasons'.)

The individual components of COM-B are defined and illustrated in Table 5.2 in relation to the target behaviour 'blending food to the right consistency'. The value of COM-B is that it enables the SLT firstly to identify exactly *what needs to happen* in order for a target behaviour to occur and, secondly, to analyze whether there is a *need for change*. For example, using the system described in Table 5.2 might be helpful for the SLT to 'diagnose' why training alone has not been fully effective and to identify some less obvious changes (such as blender availability and time) that could make the difference in safe swallowing practice.

Following the behavioural diagnosis, the speech and language therapist can more easily identify interventions that are appropriate to bring about

Table 5.2 COM-B components.

COM-B components	What needs to happen for the target behaviour to occur?	Is there a need for change?
Physical capability Physical skill, strength or stamina.	Have the physical skill to use blender.	No – all staff know how to use blender.
Psychological capability Knowledge or psychological skills, strength or stamina to engage in the necessary mental processes.	Know how much to blend different types of food to achieve correct consistency.	Change needed – staff uncertain about consistencies/national descriptors.
Physical opportunity Opportunity afforded by the environment involving time, resources, locations, cues, physical 'affordance'.	Have blender available; have time to blend food.	Change needed – staff under pressure to 'get meals out' and report they do not always have time to blend food fully. Blender is sometimes not washed up.
Social opportunity Opportunity afforded by interpersonal influences, social cues and cultural norms that influence the way we think about and see things.	See others using blender.	Change needed – see above, staff not consistent in practice.
Reflective motivation Reflective processes including plans (self-conscious intentions) and evaluations (beliefs about what is good and bad).	Hold beliefs that blending food helps to avoid aspiration.	No change needed – staff aware that modified diet supports swallowing.
Automatic motivation Automatic processes involving emotional reactions, desires (wants and needs), impulses, inhibitions, drive states and reflex responses.	Have established routines.	Change needed to establish routine and habit formation for blending food at every meal.
Behavioural diagnosis of the relevant COM-B components	Change needed in psychological capability, physical opportunity, social opportunity, automatic motivation.	

behaviour change. For example, education is particularly appropriate for enhancing psychological capability whilst persuasion can increase motivation and environmental restructuring can increase opportunity.

Specific behaviour change techniques can be thought of as the smallest 'active ingredients' of behaviour change and should be selected based on the behavioural diagnosis. Michie et al. (2013) have collated a taxonomy of behaviour change techniques (BCCTv1). Version 1 consists of 93 separate techniques organized into 16 groups: goals and planning; feedback and monitoring; social support; shaping knowledge; natural consequences; comparison of behaviour; association; repetition and substitution; comparison of outcomes; reward and threat; regulation; antecedents; identity; scheduled consequences; self-belief; and covert learning. Interestingly, in relation to ideas discussed in Chapter 4, the authors note that version 2 of the taxonomy will contain an additional category of 'enhancing positive emotions'.

The final steps described in the BCW are identifying modes of delivery (e.g., face-to-face or remotely; individually or in a group) and policy category (e.g., producing guidelines or providing a service). For the individual speech and language therapist, the highly detailed steps described in the BCW may be impractical to undertake for each client on their caseload. However, it is easy to see its potential value when designing services, as the time taken to perform detailed analysis of what behaviours are best targeted in intervention and precisely how to intervene is likely to be worth the time investment and result in a more effective (and cost-effective) service. Nevertheless, an SLT can helpfully make use of elements of the BCW when working with individual clients, particularly the core COM-B system itself, to focus their thinking about what is required and what needs to change in order for a given behaviour to happen.

Therapy as behaviour change technique

So far in this chapter, we have considered behaviour change models and techniques as if they were an 'add-on' – albeit an important one – to our 'usual' therapy activities. The work of Michie and colleagues in developing their behaviour change taxonomy has been valuable in providing a lens through which speech and language therapists can conceptualize very many therapy activities as behaviour change techniques in themselves. This is not to deny the existence or value of other things that an SLT might do, such as facilitating open discussion, listening and empathising, as discussed in Chapters 2 and

6. However, if we return to the definition of behaviour at the beginning of this chapter as a 'physical event in the body controlled by the brain', we can see that the endeavour of the SLT is indeed mainly concerned with this for, even when working with clients at the most psychological level (exploring the self-concept, working with attitudes and so on), it is ultimately for the

Table 5.3 Behaviour change techniques in speech and language therapy (Rees, 2016 [communication]). Reproduced with permission.

BCT	Definition	SLT example
Instruction on how to perform the behaviour.	Advise or agree on how to perform the behaviour.	In helping a child to produce /f/, tell them where to place their top teeth and ask them to blow. Instruct a client on how to perform vocal warm-ups.
Demonstration of the behaviour.	Provide an observable sample of the performance of the behaviour, directly in person or indirectly, e.g., via film, pictures, for the person to aspire to or imitate (includes **Modelling**),	Ask two children in a class, who have good social skills, to role-play a scenario where one makes a positive remark (e.g., Hey, nice trainers) and the other responds graciously (e.g., Thanks, mate). This would be for the benefit of other children in the same class who have difficulty accepting giving and receiving compliments. Demonstrate vocal warm-ups to a client.
Feedback on behaviour	Monitor and provide feedback on performance of the behaviour (e.g., form, frequency, duration, intensity),	Providing specific feedback on what has improved and/or what needs to be modified. Example: "Great – you remembered to say the /k/."
Feedback on outcome of behaviour	Monitor and provide feedback on the outcome of performance of the behaviour,.	Providing the required response – thus providing feedback that the behaviour has been performed correctly. Example: "You looked at me the whole time I was telling you the story so I thought you were interested and wanted to carry on." Pointing to 'key' out of two pictures of 'key' and 'tea' (when previously you pointed to 'tea' when the child was trying to say 'key').

purpose of bringing about a physical change, be this speaking more loudly for a patient with PD; using /k/ instead of /t/ when shown a key for the child who is fronting; or engaging in a situation that has long been avoided for the young adult who stammers.

From October to December 2016, a set of articles in *Bulletin*, the professional publication of the Royal College of Speech and Language Therapists, discussed the application of behaviour change theory and techniques within speech and language therapy practice, education and research (Rees, Wood, & Cavin, 2016; Stringer & Toft, 2016a, 2016b). Rachel Rees and colleagues explain how students are asked to identify their interventions in terms of the specific behaviour change techniques included in BCTTv1 (Michie et al., 2013). The advantage of this is that it provides a common terminology for speech and language therapists to draw on when they are describing what they are doing during therapy, and is also a helpful way of encouraging students to think about the therapeutic value (to change behaviour) of the specific activities they choose. Table 5.3 illustrates speech and language therapy practice examples of behaviour change techniques (Rees, 2016 [personal communication]; Rees et al., 2016).

In the context of research, identifying the behaviour change techniques that make up interventions holds promise for complex interventions such as those that typify speech and language therapy. Within evidence-based practice, the emphasis tends to be on outcomes rather than process. An intervention might be described in more or less detailed terms but there is usually limited attempt to unpick the components of therapy to understand whether or how specific aspects contribute to the outcomes in question. As Stringer and Toft (2016a) point out, this should be of interest to speech and language therapists because it is common practice to adapt therapy protocols, for example to meet the needs of specific clients or because they are working within resource constraints. The Medical Research Council has stated in guidelines for designing and evaluating complex interventions that the intervention process should be evaluated alongside outcomes.

One of the first attempts to do this in a speech and language therapy context has been the work of Fiona Johnson and colleagues (Johnson, Best, Beckley, Maxim, & Beeke, 2016). They investigated the mechanisms of change within conversational therapy for people with aphasia (Better Conversations with Aphasia: http://www.ucl.ac.uk/betterconversations/aphasia). They analyzed video and interview data from eight people with aphasia and their conversation partners and used the COM-B model to identify and categorize mechanisms of change in the context of capability, opportunity and motivation (Johnson et al., 2016). They then identified 16 reliably agreed behaviour change techniques associated with the BCA intervention, based on BCTTv1. These included goal setting, self-monitoring of outcomes, demonstration of behaviour, prompts and cues and social reward (Hibbard, Mahoney, Stockard, & Tusler, 2005). Work is continuing in this area. Nazlie and Stringer (2017) reported on a project being developed to use video tagging technology to support identification of behaviour change techniques used during therapy to enhance the learning of student speech and language therapists.

Patient activation and health coaching

With the increasing emphasis on the role of self-management during the past few years, the concept of 'patient activation' has started to generate wide interest. Patient activation is defined as "an individual's knowledge, skill and confidence for managing their health and healthcare" (Hibbard et al., 2005). It has many overlaps with ideas that have already been discussed in this chapter. For example, 'knowledge and skill' has much in common with psychological and physical capabilities as described in the COM-B model and 'confidence' seems to echo the notion of self-efficacy although, according to Hibbard and Gilburt, it is a more generalized concept. The authors do recognize, however, that activation draws on constructs such as self-efficacy and readiness to change. In a report for The Kings Fund, Hibbard and Gilburt (2014, p.7) note that individuals who have low levels of activation are, amongst other things, more likely to feel overwhelmed with the task of managing their health, feel unconfident in their ability to have a positive effect on their own health, and have limited problem-solving skills. It is then not difficult to see that, for clients with low levels of activation, a 'downward spiral' can be set up with experiences of failure resulting in further reductions of confidence and feelings of being overwhelmed.

A number of studies investigating activation in people with long-term conditions have found that higher patient activations scores are associated with greater adherence to treatment, monitoring health conditions and obtaining regular care (see Hibbard & Gilburt, 2014, for an overview of these). Research suggests that activation is associated with better health outcomes, lower care costs and a better patient experience, regardless of factors such as socio-economic status, age or culture (Hibbard & Gilburt, 2014). Whilst, to date, there have been no studies specifically investigating patient activation in population with speech, language and communication needs, Solasky, Mackenzie, Wegener, & Riley (2008) found that health behaviour counselling increased patient activation leading to higher levels of adherence to physical therapy following back surgery. A further interesting finding of this study was that activation did not increase for around one-third of participants who received counselling with the most common reason for this being identified as low self-efficacy due to lack of knowledge and support.

Other studies have also demonstrated that patient activation is modifiable. Supporting clients to gain new skills ('mastery'), supporting changes in the environment, health coaching and education classes have been areas of focus, revisiting many themes already seen in this chapter. Importantly, Hibbard and Gilburt (2014) note that not all clients are likely to be able to benefit from all types of intervention. For example, less activated patients are less likely to take advantage of, say, educational programmes on offer (Hibbard & Green, 2011). It is these 'hard to reach' populations that are often the greatest concern to speech and language therapists. For example, a service that offers parent training programmes to support parents of children with speech or language difficulties may find that it is only parents who already have relatively high levels of activation that engage with them. Therefore, in a similar way to the TTM, patient activation emphasizes the importance of tailoring interventions appropriately to the patient's level of activation. For example, the SLT working with clients with low levels of activation (which perhaps can be seen as analogous to the 'pre-contemplation' stage of the TTM) might take a 'health coaching' approach, outlined below, focusing on increasing self-awareness of current behaviour and building confidence by identifying small steps, enabling the client to build success. Again, as we noted particularly in relation to the COM-B model outlined earlier in the chapter, considerations such as increasing activation are not just important – or, indeed, most important – at an individual client–therapist level, but also need to be considered at the level of service design in an era when economic sustainability and value for money are key considerations.

Health coaching

Health coaching is becoming an influential approach to encouraging self-management and patient activation, particularly with individuals who have chronic or multiple health conditions. Important aspects of health coaching

Box 5.4 Supporting behaviour change

Jeanette

Jeanette is a single Mum living in the outskirts of a northern city. Her son, Callum, is aged 2.5. Jeanette tries her best but struggles to cope at times and there has been some involvement of social services. Callum can be difficult at times; he doesn't sleep well and often has serious tantrums. He uses very few words and usually points if he wants something or tries to get it himself. Jeanette gets exhausted as she doesn't sleep much either. She tries to catch some sleep during the day whilst Callum watches the TV. Jeanette's social worker has told her that she must attend the local Children's Centre where a speech and language therapist runs sessions advising parents on how to promote talking. She has said that if Jeanette doesn't go, it may result in a referral to the Courts. Jeanette can't see the point but reluctantly agrees because she wants to avoid a court order.

In your role as SLT at the Centre:

1. Thinking about the TTM, what 'stage' do you think Jeanette might be at?
2. From the information you have, what behavioural diagnosis do you reach, using the COM-B model?
3. How could you support the change process when you work with Jeanette?

Hayley

Hayley is a single Mum living on the outskirts of Bradford. Her son, Jacob, is aged 2.5. Jacob can be a handful and Hayley struggles to cope sometimes. About two months ago, she saw an advert for a drop-in run by a speech and language therapist at the local Children's Centre. Hayley thought it might be a good idea to go because she has noticed that Jacob is hardly using any words and doesn't seem to understand much. He often has tantrums and Hayley wondered if it might be related. She has been going along to the Centre for quite a few weeks and the SLT has given her lots of advice. Hayley struggles to put a lot of it into practice. She is supposed to play with Jacob instead of letting him watch the TV in the evenings but letting him watch is the only chance she gets to have a break and catch up with her friends so she doesn't always manage it. She tries to read to Jacob when she puts him to bed except when 'Eastenders' is on.

In your role as SLT at the Centre:

1. Thinking about the TTM, what 'stage' do you think Hayley might be at?
2. From the information you have, what behavioural diagnosis do you reach, using the COM-B model?
3. How could you support the change process when you work with Hayley, using ideas discussed within this chapter?

include working with clients to identify their goals, to engage in learning about how to achieve those goals, and to use self-monitoring of behaviours to increase accountability. The interpersonal relationship with the coach, a health professional trained in various aspects of behaviour change theory and strategies, is emphasized (Wolever et al., 2013). Thus, many of the ideas already discussed within this chapter are relevant to a health coaching approach. Reported benefits of health coaching for patients include: more effective consultations which are tailored to the patients' needs; expectations and readiness to change; changes to patient expectations; motivation and confidence to self-manage; setting more effective and realistic goals; creating shared responsibility; and improved health outcomes (Health Coaching for Behaviour Change Interim Progress Report, 2013, p.5; https://eoeleadership.hee.nhs.uk/sites/default/files/1404813191_LmkH_health_coaching_interim_progress_report.pdf).

McDowell (2014) describes a model for developing health-coaching skills that has been used to train health professionals including GPs, nurses, occupational therapists, physiotherapists and dieticians as well as speech and language therapists. The model combines three elements. Firstly, the knowledge and skills of professionals, including both specific content knowledge (for example, how to differentially diagnose a phonological disorder and verbal dyspraxia) as well as skills such as problem solving and building therapeutic relationships. Secondly, there are principles and models from health psychology such as those described in this chapter. Finally, there are skills and techniques that are more usually associated with performance coaching, although containing ideas which will be familiar to speech and language therapists in other contexts such as the use of scaling, also used in Solution Focused Brief Therapy (see Chapter 6) but also models of coaching that may be less familiar such as TGROW (Downey, 2003). It is in many ways similar to other models used in counselling and coaching such as Egan's Skilled Helper (Egan, 2009) and involves establishing the topic (T), setting the goals (G), understanding current reality (R), exploring options (O) and agreeing a way forward (W).

Conclusions

For speech and language therapy to be effective, clients need to undertake specific actions such as to practise exercises or alter their way of communicating with their child. It is of critical importance that clients do these things because, if they do not, even the most well-evidenced speech and language therapy interventions will be ineffective. Strategies for supporting behaviour change are likely to become increasingly important as the policy focus continues to shift towards self-management. A number of theories as well as practical ideas for supporting adherence to therapy and behaviour change have been discussed in this chapter. As Michie's identification of approaching 100 separate theories of behaviour change illustrates, this can only scratch the surface. Within the few ideas discussed here, however, it is noticeable that there are similarities and overlaps, as well as some differences, between the models and techniques described. One of the most practical and effective things that the SLT can do is to support clients to adhere to advice given, and to help them understand and remember it. It is important to be aware of the client's readiness for change and to select an intervention accordingly; expecting the client to act when they are only in the early stages of contemplating change is likely to result in failure. The concept of self-efficacy is a common theme throughout many models of behaviour change. Important sources of self-efficacy are mastery experiences and learning from others. Another important strategy is trying to ensure that performing a new behaviour requires as little self-regulatory 'effort' as possible; one way of doing this is to increase the automaticity by helping clients form a detailed plan of when, where and how they will carry out the activities. Detailed analysis of the factors that influence behaviour change can reveal ideas for actions that might otherwise not be considered. Recent developments from the field of performance coaching are being applied in health settings to support the self-management agenda.

Finally, this chapter has focused on ideas about behaviour change and self-management. Although self-management is often talked about as being linked with – or even the same thing as – person care, we believe that it is worth reflecting, from the perspective of personal values and preferences, on how the ideas presented in this chapter interact with the ideas of person-centred care and the therapeutic alliance that were discussed in Chapter 2.

6 Therapeutic processes

Introduction

The previous chapters have considered a range of ideas and frameworks in psychology which can be applied in speech and language therapy practice. Common themes have included the development of therapeutic relationships with clients, seeking to understand their perspective and supporting the process of change. In order to develop further understanding of psychological ideas, it seems important to consider the application and practical use of this knowledge. This chapter focuses on emotional wellbeing in the client, and considers therapeutic behaviours and approaches based in social and counselling psychology applied to the practice of speech and language therapy. It aims to explore the relationship between the emotional, attitudinal and cognitive aspects of the individual in therapy and offers guidelines for relevant practice.

It is important to discuss the specific professional areas where counselling is pertinent to the professional interaction and there are some useful distinctions to make. 'Counselling' might be considered to take two forms. Directive counselling refers to giving advice about a specific condition, such as advice on swallowing techniques. Many speech and language therapy students feel 'at home' in this territory, which casts the therapist in the role of 'expert' who will try to 'fix' the problem that brings. On the other hand, non-directive counselling offers the client an opportunity to talk through attitudes and feelings about a situation in a nonjudgmental context, working out their own solutions to problems in a supportive atmosphere.

For some groups, such as people who stammer or individuals with functional voice disorders, counselling is quite likely to form a core part of the therapeutic activity. Dalton (1994) discusses the importance of providing counselling for children and adults who stammer, taking into account the impact of stammering on their whole life experience. She made particular note of the adolescent years where stammering may be especially significant. Dalton refers to this as a time when speech really 'mattered'. The preoccupation and anxiety around speaking impacts so greatly upon the day-to-day life of the individual that counselling may be a central part of enabling improvement. In other contexts, such as individuals with acquired conditions including brain injury, stroke and neurodegenerative disorders, there may be a significant range of physical and emotional challenges including communication difficulties. In this case, although not a core aspect of therapy, there may be times when it is important to spend clinical time on enabling the individual to understand their condition more fully and for them to work out ways of managing it in the future. Counselling may also be relevant for the adolescent with any type or communication impairment or the parent of a child with a disability. As Shames (2006), notes, you do not relinquish the speech and language therapy role but it may be necessary to delay some aspects of therapy in order to respond to sensitive matters which arise spontaneously in the therapy time. For example, the person who is aphasic may be concentrating on word-finding activities, but one of the prompt pictures reminds him of a distressing aspect of the impact of his stroke and he may need to focus on his feelings about that.

Rollin (1987) described a wide scope of application to counselling for people with speech and language difficulties. Clearly, the profile of the communication impairment and the individual's response to it will influence the way the emotional needs of the client are addressed. Various clinical contexts may have different requirements, where the client experiences challenges which indirectly impact on the communication difficulty. For example, loss of mobility from stroke may create social isolation for an individual, therefore

---

Box 6.1 Help outside speech and language therapy?

Kathy and Mark had their son, Jamie, when they were 19 when they were both struggling to find work. Although they had managed to rent a flat, and eventually obtained some low-paid work, Kathy had not been able to continue working because the costs of child care for Jamie were so high. Even with benefits, it was still too costly. Her relationship with Mark deteriorated around this time and they eventually separated with Mark moving out to live in another town. Kathy found this a very difficult time and although she had parents and a sister nearby she struggled with the sole responsibility of Jamie and the cost of living. She felt lonely and isolated. Jamie was late in developing language and during the speech and language therapy sessions she attended with him, she found that she could talk easily to the speech and language therapist.

Kathy's situation did have an impact upon Jamie but her difficulties needed more specialized support and the therapist was concerned to help her find guidance and counselling in relation to the broader aspects of managing her life. Following some discussion, the therapist found help for Kathy through a social worker.

indirectly limiting opportunities for communication practice. The individual may benefit from a non-directive counselling approach to enable them to create improvements or change. There may also be clinical situations where the client or carer or parent bring up material which is a cause of concern but not directly related to the communication difficulty; for example, the single parent may want to talk about the impact of her situation on her child's development, as outlined in Box 6.1.

Individuals who are offered counselling will usually receive this from counsellors who might have been trained to focus on a specific theoretical position, such as client-centred counselling (Rogers, 1951) or cognitive-behavioural therapy. In addition to these services, which may be private or within the NHS, there are also contexts where there is a role for some forms of counselling across a range of professions. Syder and Levy (1998) describe this as not taking a primary role, but a situation about which it is professionally acceptable to use the term 'using counselling skills' (Bond, 1993). Examples from medicine, nursing and the police could be where, during the course of an interaction, an individual becomes distressed and may need counselling, such as a patient expressing concerns about a condition, a patient describing difficulties in coping, or a person in a police station requiring support about an incident. Nelson-Jones (2015) uses the term 'helpers' to describe professionals and others who use counselling skills as part of other primary roles and who are trained in counselling skills but are not professionally accredited counsellors or psychotherapists. Thus, counselling may be used as part of the scope of practice but is not central or key to the professional activity and is not part of the name of the profession. The use of counselling in the speech and language therapy context would reflect this type of activity. A distinction is therefore made between being an accredited counsellor and another professional making intentional use of specific interpersonal counselling skills in certain contexts. The guidelines refer to the use of counselling skills as enhancing the professional role whilst still acting within the primary role of a speech and language therapist. Thus, the use of counselling skills is made relevant as part of the scope of practice.

It is important to consider the role and purpose of non-directive counselling skills with reference to speech and language therapy clients who may be a special case within the population of those who need counselling. Not only are many of these clients coping with communication difficulties that affect everyday life, in addition they may have limited means of expressing feelings.

For most speakers, talking through problems is a generally accepted way of coping; with severe communication impairment this may be much more difficult. The speech and language therapist has excellent skills for listening and facilitating and may be more able to communicate about feelings and concerns than other health care professionals. As Shames (2006) said:

> "Having a communication disability does not immunise a person from the problems of everyday living, but rather does just the opposite. It targets such a person and makes him or her even more vulnerable to emotional problems. Therefore, communication problems, by definition, must include these interactive and emotional components, and therefore demand clinical and therapeutic attention."
>
> *Shames, 2006, p.xvi*

Therapists may often feel uncertain about how to manage a client who has issues which are causing distress. If the therapeutic approach requires a specific form of language therapy, then a therapist may be anxious about using therapy time to respond to emotional distress. It is clearly a concern for many therapists and some research has shown that this issue can be of critical importance. Brumfitt (2006) in a survey of 173 speech and language therapists who were members of the British Aphasiology Society found that 97% of participants stated that psychosocial aspects were either important or very important to the overall management of their clients. Ninety-five percent stated that the psychosocial status was important or very important to the overall outcome of their intervention. Thus, there is clear evidence that in the context of aphasia the matter of responding to distress does cause concern for the speech and language therapist. This needs to be acknowledged and consideration given to how a therapist might proceed with this additional role in the scope of practice. In a recent study, Shrubsole, Worrall, Power and O'Connor (2016) reported a systematic review of stroke in Australia and one outcome was for further work to increase understanding about the role of counselling in the management of that condition.

Holland and Nelson (2014) have an interesting discussion in their book on the role of counselling with people with communication difficulties. For many speech and language therapists this role may feel an easy transition but for others it may be challenging. Many therapists are concerned about their level of skill, and the role of universities in developing these skills in students is an important one to acknowledge.

What are useful behaviours for speech and language therapists to develop in relation to providing some level of counselling support? Holland and Nelson (2014) have some useful ideas in relation to characteristics of successful clinicians. That is, what attitudes and behaviours are useful to this role? Holland states that it is important to reveal yourself to others (that is, be clear about who you are), and be in touch with your feelings and capabilities (know your strengths in the clinical setting and let others see these). Additionally, always aim to see each person as unique. All differences or challenges faced in the clinic are learning experience, not threats or signals for conflict. Holland and Nelson further recommend that the therapist understands the client for who they are, not how the therapist wishes them to be. And finally, the therapist must understand that clients are responsible for their own behaviour; the therapist can guide and respond and suggest, but ultimately the client makes the decision whether or not to move forward and respond (Holland & Nelson, 2007, p.68). These ideas echo many of the themes we discussed in Chapter 2 when we considered what it means to 'be therapeutic'.

It is important for the speech and language therapist to understand and learn about the skills involved in counselling and to be able to understand how to apply these to various clinical situations. However, it is also important to recognize that the client comes to us for speech and language therapy and not for counselling, and we need to be mindful of our role and its boundaries. In discussing the application of counselling when working with people who stammer, Turnbull (2000) refers to the Dual Process Model of Loss (Stroebe & Schut, 1999, cited in Turnbull, 2000). The model describes two types of coping in bereavement: loss oriented and restoration oriented. Turnbull suggests that clients who stammer may spend the early part of therapy enmeshed in loss or suffering oriented processes. The therapist needs to recognize and explore this with the client but be prepared to refer him or her for counselling if they are unable to then develop a restoration-oriented focus, for example, if there continue to be pervasive negative emotions. It can easily be seen that this would be a useful concept to apply when working with many clients. Turnbull also discusses the issue of competence and credibility; the speech and language therapist needs to be aware of his or her own skills and refer on to a counsellor or other SLT if they feel they do not have sufficient skills to undertake a counselling approach with the client at the level needed.

Basic skills in counselling

Although approaches to counselling may vary according to different theoretical frameworks, there is a recognition that the three conditions of a counselling relationship – first identified by Rogers (1951) – provide a strong basis or starting point (http://counsellingtutor.com/counselling-approaches/person-centred-approach-to-counselling/carl-rogers-core-conditions/). In order to show acceptance of the client, Rogers believed that the counsellor should display attitudes which allow the client to feel valued. These are described as 'core conditions'. Rogers believed that the core conditions enable the therapist to demonstrate acceptance of the client, valuing them as a human being with worth. This safe environment supports the individual to realize their own potential and begin to find their own answers to problems.

Congruence or transparency: This refers to the counsellor being open and genuine with the client as opposed to revealing little of their own personality. According to Rogers this congruence will enable the client to be more receptive to a deeper conversation with the counsellor as it will be easier to feel trust and talk more easily if the counsellor is open.

Unconditional positive regard: Rogers believed that for people to grow and fulfil their potential it is important that they are valued as themselves rather than being seen as a distant individual who can be manipulated. The therapist has a deep and genuine regard for the client which allows the client to develop and respond to the therapeutic conversation. It is intended that the client is valued for who they are rather than being judged for who they are. This may have potential difficulties as the client may reveal issues which are of concern to the counsellor. These may be risky or socially inappropriate behaviours or there may be features of the client which remind the counsellor of their own experience, thus making the relationship more difficult.

Empathic understanding: Rogers described empathy as the counsellor's ability to enter into the feelings, thoughts and experiences of another and to understand what the client is feeling. It is a state of perceiving and relating to another person's feelings and needs without the need to blame, give advice or repair the situation.

Counselling microskills

Developing and using a range of counselling skills, sometimes referred to as microskills, is an important part of the speech and language therapist's skills.

They support the development of the therapeutic relationship and help to create and convey to clients the core conditions described above. Some of the most valuable skills are described below. Although the prospect may be rather unappealing, it is worth noting that having the opportunity to practise these skills and record yourself on video can provide an invaluable insight into your body language, facial expressions and verbal 'tics'! The opportunity to watch others is also extremely useful; observing what others do and say in response to challenging therapy encounters, and noticing what works and what does not, enables the speech and language therapist to build up his or her own repertoire of phases and questions. On the whole, however, there is no substitute for trying things out yourself, perhaps with a friend to colleague, particularly with some of the more specific counselling techniques that are described a little later in the chapter.

Attending: appropriate seating/open posture/appropriate eye contact: It is important that the client feels the therapist is listening carefully. Shames (2006) notes that attending closely to what the client says can communicate a positive experience and enable the client to feel that what he or she says has value and is worth listening to. Various nonverbal messages can be unintentionally communicated if the therapist does not show good nonverbal listening behaviours. For example, if the therapist avoids eye contact and appears to be looking even minimally away from the client this may cause uncertainty and insecure feelings about whether the client feels able to continue confiding. Thus, the seating position and nonverbal behaviours of the therapist should be appropriate and open and relaxed, enabling the client to feel comfortable. It is interesting that Holland (2007) recommends full body listening, where the therapist should use culturally acceptable nonverbal behaviours in listening. Holland (2007) emphasizes the importance of being sensitive to the cultural norms in this way.

Listening and giving encouragers to talk; nonverbal and verbal: Good listening behaviour will include non-intrusive listening, allowing the client to feel comfortable about talking without fear of constant interruption from the therapist. The therapist must show that listening is taking place and this may involve a degree of appropriate, but not over-intense, concentration on what the client is saying, following up where necessary if the client says something which is not clear. This is usually referred to as active listening. The therapist can use nonverbal and verbal listening behaviours such as nodding appropriately and using non-linguistic interventions such as 'mmm'. Appropriate use of 'yes/no/I see' can also be included here. However, Shames (2006) warns against the use of too many stereotypical behaviours which may become repetitive and boring if they are used continuously. There is the risk of the therapist appearing less genuine and interested if the same behaviours are repeated. Shames refers to the problems with 'head bobbing' throughout the interaction. Recommendations for a varied use of nonverbal and verbal responders are made and this will permit the client to feel that the listening is more real and a genuine response. Some examples include, "I see/I understand/Could you say a little more about…". Silence can also be a very powerful tool here, and simply waiting can often elicit valuable insights from clients; many students as well as more experienced therapists struggle with the idea of silence but the skill of *not* saying something is one that is worth developing.

Probing skills: closed and open questions and funnelling: Both closed and open questions play an important role in the counselling conversation. It is important to use a variety of these types of question in order to develop the relationship and understanding of the client. There will be different times when either open or closed questioning is appropriate. Shames (2006) also recommends the use of 'instructions' as opposed to questions which

---

Box 6.2 Questions and probing

Closed questions: very specific, fact-seeking questions

    "Do you want a cup of tea?"

    "Do you have difficulties getting to sleep at night?"

    "Do you notice difficulties with hearing what others say?"

Open questions: questions which allow choice in the answer

    "How have you been since last week?"

    "What sort of things do you like to do at the weekend?"

    "What types of speaking situations are most challenging for you?"

'Instructions' or an invitation to talk (Shames, 2006)

    "Tell me why you are here today."

    "Tell me about your accident."

may make the client more comfortable and find it easier to talk. Box 6.2 shows some examples of types of questions suggested by Shames (2006).

In addition, funnelling is a technique which is used to focus down on the client's answers so that each question becomes more restrictive at each stage. Thus, the therapist starts with open questions and moves to closed or the other way round. For example:

"Tell me about your stammering." (very open question)

"What are the challenges?"

"Are there any times when it is worse?"

"Have you tried speech and language therapy?"

"Did the slowed speech technique help you?" (very specific question).

The questions in this example become more restrictive, starting with open questions which allow for very broad answers where the individual can say what seems most relevant, but at each stage the questions become more focused and the answers become more restrictive or closed. The aim of funnelling is to help clients focus on their concerns by narrowing down to specific aspects.

Empathic skills: reflecting/paraphrasing/summarizing: Empathy is a personal quality which some people naturally have and which can be further developed through practice. Do you have empathy? It is most likely that you do because you are interested in the psychology of people. When you read a newspaper article about the experience of an individual, read a book or watch a film you are likely to enter into the world of the key individuals in the story and feel some of the impact of their experiences. To a certain extent this is the same when working with clients. The client describes their situation and the therapist empathizes with the situation by having the capacity to engage with the experience. Often the therapist can show empathy to the client by summarizing what has just been said. This may be valuable for the client who may feel their situation is closely understood. An example of this might be where the client talks about his experiences since his head injury and the therapist summarizes by saying: *"So, I can see that the injury has made you much less confident than you used to be and this has led to you feeling much more isolated. I can see that this is difficult for you right now."*

This capacity or skill is not the same as understanding an individual because you have the same shared experiences. It is most likely that you may not have a shared experience with your client. Your client may be of a different generation, and have a medical or psychological condition which you have not experienced yourself. Therefore, empathy is what you need. You need to be able to enter into the experience of the individual, imagine what their experience must be like and thus be able to use this to work out a strategy for helping the individual.

Applying counselling skills in speech and language therapy

Having discussed in general terms the counselling role of the speech and language therapist and considered some of the basic skills involved, three specific applications of counselling are considered below: managing emotional distress; working with parents and children; and working with groups.

Managing emotional distress

The thought of managing emotional distress when working with a client is one that is often difficult for staff or students to feel comfortable with or confident about. In a speech and language therapy context there will be a variety of situations where clients become distressed, such as in a stroke unit where clients are in the early stages of recovery or in situations with parents coping with a child with a range of disabilities. When people cry, they may have a variety of feelings about doing it. For example, it may feel quite comfortable to cry in front of your family but it uncomfortable to cry in front of a stranger. It may also work the other way for some people. For example, it may be easier to cry in front of a stranger because you may feel you are not burdening that person with your problem; whereas you may feel your family is already burdened

---

Box 6.3 Holding silence

Next time a friend is talking to you about something that is worrying them, make a conscious decision to pause and hold the silence when they stop speaking. Notice what happens. Does your friend say something more? How did you feel?

with your problem and you do not wish to make them feel worse. It depends entirely on the individual circumstance. Some people may cry on hearing any sort of bad news whether it affects them or not; others may only respond with crying if the news directly affects them.

Two understandings of crying may need to be remembered for clinical work:

1. Crying may release feelings and allow patients to unburden themselves; thus being able to move on and look for solutions, and cope with the problem better.

2. Crying may feel like a 'loss of face'. The individual may feel they have made themselves look 'inadequate' and be embarrassed.

This is, however, very dependent on the circumstances and the individual. For the speech and language therapist, it is important to be aware that your clients may cry and may have differing feelings about doing so. There may be cultural or possibly gender factors involved in this; for example, different cultures may have varying expectations of whether it is socially appropriate to cry in a public setting. Society also has varying agreement about whether it is appropriate for men to cry. In addition, there may be a range of views about whether it is socially acceptable for a male patient to cry in front of a female therapist. This may also be influenced by the condition itself. For example, post-acute stroke conditions may cause a great deal of emotion as the individual starts to recover from the major impact of the stroke. Crying may also have neurological cause, such as in pathological crying or emotional lability which is recognized in many acquired neurological conditions. Remember too, that if clients cry, they may not be able to tell the therapist *why* they are crying because of their communication impairment. As a therapist, you may have to make guesses.

Barton (2010) discusses the importance of enabling staff to manage emotional distress in a healthcare setting and offers advice, summarized in Box 6.4.

Pathological crying

Pathological crying (PC) is a poorly understood neurological condition, usually associated with acquired neurological damage or degeneration. It is often referred to as 'pseudobulbar affect', where the threshold for laughing or crying is lowered so that the individual appears to laugh or cry inappropriately.

Box 6.4 Managing emotional distress

1. Listening to the patient is perhaps the most crucial skill. This is not always easy, but by using a combination of verbal and nonverbal methods of communication this can be made easier.

2. Let the patient know that you have heard what they are 'saying' and that you have understood. If you have not understood what the patient is trying to communicate to you, it is important to acknowledge this with the patient, and suggest that you will need to do some more exploration of what the problem is.

3. Try to concentrate on what the patient is trying to communicate to you. Focus on how the patient is behaving as well as what they are saying.

4. Remember that if a patient is distressed or is crying, it is important for the member of staff to acknowledge this distress and not to avoid it or shy away from it. The last thing that patients want to hear when they are upset is that 'everything will be all right'. Of course, patients do want reassurance, but they also want to have their distress acknowledged and validated.

5. Remember to make eye contact with the patient, and to try to keep an open body posture, so that the patient knows that you are interested in what they are trying to communicate to you. (Barton, 2009, p.148).

Parvizi et al. (2006) define pathological crying as "episodes of laughing or crying, without an apparent motivating stimulus, or in response to stimuli that would not have elicited such an emotional response before the onset of their underlying neurological condition". Emotional outbursts may be exaggerated in nature, or can in fact seem to wholly contradict the emotional prompt or context. For example, a patient with PC may laugh uncontrollably when frustrated or angry, or cry unexpectedly during an everyday mundane conversation. These outbursts do not reflect the underlying mood of the patient.

Typically, these behaviours may be seen in acute stroke units where the individual is in the early stages of recovery. Anderson (1997) reported that post-stroke pathological crying is more common than generally understood and quotes studies where 20% of patients during the first year post-stroke have shown these symptoms. In severe cases, Anderson (1997) reports episodes of post-stroke pathological crying as occurring up to 100 times a day. These may be very difficult symptoms for the individual to cope with. The symptoms

Table 6.1 Differences between pathological crying and depression (Parvizi et al., 2006).

Pathological crying	Depression
Emotion does not reflect patient's real mood	Emotion reflects real feelings/mood
Crying not associated with physical symptoms of depression	Crying may be associated with symptoms like decreased energy, poor concentration, feelings of helplessness
Crying episodes usually short in duration	Sadness experienced over time

may impact on social interaction and family members may find this difficult. Furthermore, potential difficulties are created for the professional in making an accurate diagnosis of true depression or pathological crying. This lack of understanding is partly due to the complex relationship between PC and depression, with confusion regarding whether the two are distinct or co-existing.

Working with children and their families

The worries and concerns a parent may have when considering how they will manage life with a child with a disability are outlined by Holland and Nelson (2014). These include concerns about whether the parent can manage to be a good parent, how they manage their time, how they discipline their child and where they can obtain advice. In addition, parents may have concerns about how they explain their child's condition to others who do not know him. Some parents may have been worried about the possibility of their child developing a communication difficulty and the confirmation of this may in some cases be a relief. For other parents, the confirmation of a communication difficulty may arouse many anxieties and concerns. For example, the diagnosis of autism can be devastating for some parents bringing about a sense of loss and grief for the longed-for child or ideal child (https://www.autism.com/understanding_advice). These parents may fear for the future, both in terms of their child's development and in relation to the rest of the family. This concept of the loss of the 'ideal' child is often referred to across the psychological and psychiatric disciplines and refers to the internal conflict parents or caretakers may experience as they parent a child who is facing a range of difficulties including disability and communication impairment. They also have to face the challenges of negotiating potential bureaucracy associated with gaining the necessary support and speech and language therapists may find themselves in the role of advocate for parents negotiating complex statutory and voluntary systems of service provision.

Holland and Nelson (2014) have two very useful chapters on the use of counselling with parents of children at risk for disability and for children and adolescents with later developing communication disorders. In a broad discussion of the needs of parents and of clients, Holland and Nelson outline strategies to help everyday coping including using the positive counselling described in PERMA (see Chapter 4). They also note the range of resources to which the speech and language therapist can direct parents, including networks and support groups as well as internet resources (see Chapter 2 for a further discussion of this).

In a very practical book Geldard, Geldard and Yin Foo (2013) present a range of psychological approaches and methods which can be used with children. This framework provides a helpful model to enhance deeper professional understanding of the child who faces difficulty. In order to proceed with therapy, Geldard et al. (2013) emphasize that there are important attributes to the child counselling relationship which must be complied with if the therapy is to be effective. Seven attributes about the relationship are listed and these are: a connecting link between the child's world and the counsellor; exclusive; safe; authentic; confidential (subject to limits); non-intrusive; and purposeful. The authors also emphasize the need for the therapist/counsellor to consider goals set for a series of sessions and to identify the different levels at which goals can be set in order to make the counselling relevant and these are described as: Level 1 Fundamental goals; Level 2 Parents' goals; Level 3 Goals formulated by the counsellor; Level 4 Child's goals.

Geldard et al. (2013) emphasize the need for the counsellor to consider the goals of the therapy from all of these perspectives. Their overall framework for looking at the role of counselling focuses on their model known as SPICC (the Sequentially Planned Integrative Counselling Model) in which they describe the 'spiral of therapeutic change' which reflects how children may move through the counselling process. The main stages are described below.

The child joins with the counsellor: Geldard et al. (2013) emphasize that the relationship between the child and the counsellor must be reciprocal. Thus, in beginning the therapy, the counsellor joins in with the child, using some joint activity such as free play allowing the child to relax and feel comfortable.

The child begins to tell their story: Depending on the context and the counsellor using appropriate skills, the child is enabled to tell their story either by speaking directly or through indirect play. An example is given of using miniature animals to represent important family relationships.

The child's awareness of issues increases: As the child tells their story, awareness of strong feelings or emotions may emerge. At this point the child may either continue to tell their story, allowing the therapy process to continue, or withdraw and choose to stop speaking.

The child deals with deflection and resistance: If the child withdraws from painful feelings in order to cope with the challenges in their life, the counsellor will need to help the child to deal with this resistance in a way which is acceptable to the child.

The child develops a different perspective or view of self: During this process the child may begin to develop a new sense of self which is based on a clearer understanding of the real events and different from the image previously acquired.

The child rehearses, experiments with and evaluates different options: The child is supported to experiment with new approaches and behaviours towards their challenging situation. This might involve a conscious decision to learn new social skills which allows the child to cope more effectively.

The child reaches resolution and moves towards more adaptive functioning: Geldard et al. (2013) describe this stage as completing the journey round the spiral of change where the child reaches some form of resolution. The child can either move into normal adaptive functioning or return to the beginning of the spiral in order to deal with new issues.

Depending on the clinical context, and the severity of the child's communication difficulty, Rollin (1987) recommends the use of family therapy and play therapy (usually requiring specially trained therapists).

Working with groups

Groups will serve different purposes for the range of communication difficulties. Some group approaches will include educational and social rehabilitation activities but others may have a wider scope and focus on emotions. In Chapter 5, the importance of self-efficacy in successful behaviour change was discussed. Groups provide an opportunity for vicarious learning (an important contributor to self-efficacy) from a credible source, that is, other people who are experiencing the same difficulties. Brown and Knox (2010) described group therapy using an interprofessional approach for people in an acute stroke rehabilitation unit. The aim of the group was to allow patients to talk about their experiences, enhance their social contacts and gain information and support from other group members. Change following attendance at the group was measured with the VASES (Brumfitt & Sheeran, 1999), the non-sexist blob tree (Wilson, 1988) and a simple questionnaire. Group members showed positive change in their VASES rating on 'confidence', 'cheerfulness', 'optimism' and 'levels of frustration'. Generally, patients positioned themselves higher up the blob tree after the group than before. The questionnaire revealed some positive satisfaction post-group therapy. It was also noted that the group members were more confident about expressing their need for help and services and were more able to participate.

Additional work reporting on groups using Solution Focused Therapy can be found in Burns (2010) where two approaches are discussed. These are single session groups set in neurological care contexts where acute stroke patients may attend as drop-in patients to talk through their experiences adjusting to stroke. Here, Burns describes a solution focused approach. In addition, Burns (2010) describes a short-term single topic group such as 'Managing Parkinson's Disease successfully' using a solution focused approach, which has helpful practical applications.

Liddle, James and Hardman (2011) discussed the role of group therapy for older children and adults who stammer arguing that there is a strong rationale for its use. Rather than focusing specifically on speech output the authors argued that groups can address affective, behavioural and cognitive responses to stammering which may help in reducing both negative thoughts and feelings and the sense of social isolation often reported by people who stammer (Yalom & Leszcz, 2005). Liddle et al. (2011) examined the current practices of speech and language therapists in the UK regarding the use of groups. Of 143 returned questionnaires, 70% of services provided some sort of group therapy but the level of provision was variable. Barriers to group therapy included lack of participants able to travel to the venues and a perception by the services that clients were not fully committed to the notion of working in groups. However, this survey highlighted important patterns of service delivery and enhanced the profession's understanding of current provision. Further work needs to be undertaken to allow therapists to consider and develop approaches which may make group therapy provisions align more closely to academic rationale. It may be that intensive residential group therapy approaches which include counselling approaches but also other activities are advisable, such as the Swindon Fluency courses for children from the age of 8 years up to the age of 17 years (http://www.thefluencytrust.org.uk).

Approaches to counselling relevant to speech and language therapy

A variety of psychological approaches have been applied to the speech and language therapy context. Their use varies widely in terms of whether the purist version of the technique is used or whether some aspects of the approach are extrapolated and applied to a specific clinical situation. The main categories of approaches to counselling are person-centred counselling, cognitive or cognitive behavioural therapies, and psychodynamic therapies. The application of the techniques from each of these approaches can be found in various speech and language therapy methodologies but the amount and type has varied greatly.

The person-centred (or client-centred) approach to counselling has developed from the work of Carl Rogers (Rogers, 1951) and represents a humanistic orientation to counselling. Person-centred counselling offers the client a relationship based on the core conditions outlined earlier in this chapter. It is a conscious process, accepts the client for what they are, permits some self-disclosure by therapist and encourages expression of feelings. The focus is mainly on the relationship between client and therapist, facilitating change through the open and trusting interactions. The counselling skills and approaches that have been outlined so far in this chapter could be broadly construed as a version of a person-centred approach.

The psychodynamic approach is based on work developed by Freud (1933) and this focuses on the ways in which the unconscious acts on how people behave and function. Freud's belief was that feelings, desires, beliefs and needs, which the individual was not consciously aware of, could influence behaviour. Psychoanalysis is the main therapy in the psychodynamic approach and its goal is to release powerful thoughts or feelings which lie inside the unconscious mind. Often these feelings are described as repressed. It makes use of the unconscious and the therapist must be opaque with no self-disclosure. One typical context for the application of psychoanalysis is in the recalling of repressed childhood memories, for example in the case of abuse in childhood. It is important to note that this type of analysis is not within the speech and language therapist's scope of practice, although some therapists do pursue further training and may apply it if registered as a psychoanalyst.

Although it is generally difficult to place this in a particular category, Personal Construct Theory and Therapy was devised by Kelly (1955) and is often considered a cognitive therapy. It is based upon the theory that individuals understand their personal world by means of a system of constructs. These constructs will develop from experience and anticipation of experience and will have individual variation in terms of what each construct means. Kelly used the philosophical term 'constructive alternativism' to underpin all of the theory. Its main premise was that there are always different ways to interpret or give meaning to an event, allowing the individual to never become trapped by the past. Every individual will have a personal set of meanings or 'constructs' and it is these meanings or constructs that the therapist works with. That is, one person may have a system of constructs about what it means to be a 'successful speaker' which may be different from another person's understanding of 'successful speaker'. The therapist would work with each client using their individual constructs of 'successful speaker' to develop new constructs leading to a changed construction of their world. Personal construct therapy (PCT) has been used when working with people who stammer (Fransella, 1972), and people who have aphasia (Brumfitt, 1984; Dalton, 1994). Kelly devised the repertory grid technique as a means of identifying an individual's core constructs and the relationship between them although, in its full form, it is quite complex

---

Box 6.5 Self-characterization

'I want you to write a character sketch of (name) just as if he/she were the principal character in a play. Write it as it might be written by a friend who knew him/her very well and very sympathetically, perhaps better than anyone could ever know him. Be sure to write it in the third person. For example, start out by saying "(name) is..."' (Kelly, 1955, p.323).

Write your own self-characterization and ask a friend to do the same. Swap what you have written and take turns exploring what each of you has written. You could ask about the experience of writing it (some people find this quite difficult whereas, for others, it is easy). Pay particular attention to what is written at the beginning and end. Does the self-characterization seem to refer to outside influences or the person's own control? It can also be interesting to probe a little into what is missing!

and time-consuming. A simpler alternative is self-characterization, in which clients are asked to write a short description of themselves (see Box 6.5).

Probably one of the most well-known and widely used counselling approaches is cognitive behavioural therapy (CBT), founded in the 1960s by Aaron Beck (1970) and based on clinical observation that patients would typically have some form of internal dialogue which was negative and self-defeating. The internal dialogue appeared to influence behaviour and therefore it was hypothesized that changing the internal 'talk' would impact upon behaviour. The therapy of CBT therefore concentrates on the thoughts, feelings, beliefs and attitudes held by the individual patient. There are two specific components of therapy and these are (1) cognitive restructuring of thinking patterns, and (2) behavioural activation where the individual overcomes barriers to participating in activities. Recent years have seen other broadly cognitive counselling approaches being used in a speech and language therapy context including Solution Focused Therapy (O'Connell, 1998), and narrative therapy. Below, some of these approaches, and their application in speech and language therapy, are outlined.

Solution focused brief therapy

Solution focused brief therapy SFBT, (O'Connell, 1998) is a form of 'brief therapy' developed in the USA in the 1980s. It has been applied to the SLT client base particularly in voice and stammering therapy. Burns (2005) describes several cases where this approach has been used successfully with clients who have different neurological conditions, such as Parkinson's Disease, stammering and stroke, and with family members of people affected. Solution focused brief therapy is practical, future oriented, and focused on change with the emphasis being on action taken by the client to bring about some sort of change in the way they respond to or manage the problem. Thus, trying out speaking situations which cause anxiety for someone who stammers may be appropriate. In a similar way to experimentation and hypothesis testing in approaches such as PCT and CBT, the client is encouraged to use a task assignment and aim to do something which differs from their typical behaviour. Planning the assignment with the client can focus the therapy away from 'tell me about the problem' to a clearer focus on creating change.

It is important to note that there are a range of clients for whom this therapy is unsuitable and these include: those needing hospitalisation for mental health problems; psychotic clients; very obsessional clients; those who have been 'sent' to therapy (i.e., not self-directed and choosing to attend); and clients who have no social contacts and remain isolated.

SFBT therapy is always relationship based and is intended to be socially interactive with the focus of the therapeutic work being on the way the client relates to others. As well as being action based, it is also detail based, ensuring that discussions between therapist and client do focus down on the detail of what the task assignments might involve. For example, if the agreed goal was for the client to practise making phone calls, the therapist would ensure that the specific components of making a call are discussed before any assignment was carried out. The therapy is also time limited in the sense that, unlike psychoanalytic approaches, it is not a long-term therapy.

One of the values of solution focused brief therapy is that it has a clear structure for the professional to follow. The broad structure is not dissimilar to that of Egan's Skilled Helper model (Egan, 1998), widely used in counselling and coaching contexts, and also very useful in speech and language therapy (exploring the current situation; helping the client establish aims and goals; helping the client develop strategies). A useful summary of the stages and skills to use in each can be found here (http://mystrongfamily.co.uk/downloads/PDFs/SFP-EasyIntroToEgan.pdf), amongst many other places on the web. SFBT is a 4-step counselling process, with an additional step compared to Egan, that of exploring the client's own attempted solution and looking for exceptions. Each step includes guidance on questions and prompts to use with the client. The steps and their basic principles are outlined below.

Step 1 Defining the problem: It is suggested that some time is spent talking about why the client has chosen to come to therapy, taking into account this will vary according to what diagnosis the client has, their age and experience and their capacity to communicate. Specific wording for some of the questions is recommended, such as the question "What would be useful for me to understand about this situation?". The purpose of this question is to encourage the client to think about the problem and then identify what the real issues are within the problem. In the speech and language context it needs to be recognized that the wording in this question may be too complex for some client groups.

Step 2 Exploring attempted solutions and finding exceptions: The purpose of this step is to help the client use their own experience to work towards finding a solution. It is useful for the client to think about how solutions were found to other challenges in the past, either those which were similar to the current concern or completely different. To facilitate further reflection on the situation, solution focused brief therapy also encourages the client to consider times when the current concern has not been a challenge, or been less of a challenge. An example might be for a voice client to report that no vocal difficulties were noted when away on holiday but that the vocal difficulties had emerged again on returning to work. This example (referred to in solution focused terms as 'exception') could be used to discuss the factors affecting this variation in the client's experience and whether anything could be learned from it.

Step 3 Setting a goal: Like speech and language therapy contexts in general, solution focused brief therapy advises working with the client to create a relevant goal. The advice is for the goal to be something which is meaningful to the client, something which is manageable and practical taking into account client lifestyle, and the goal should be stated in positive terms, not negative. Thus, a goal which stated "I will aim to stop getting nervous about speaking to strangers" would be seen as less helpful than a goal which stated "I will aim to practise speaking to strangers every day for the next three weeks". A typical prompt question at this stage might be: "Based on your understanding of the problem, what would be a reasonable goal to set for yourself?" Taking into account the communication difficulties, it may be necessary for the therapist to provide some additional linguistic structure and support in order to enable the client to achieve this aim.

Step 4 Generating ways to reach the goal: Once a goal has been agreed it is essential to spend time with the client working out a method which will allow the client to reach the goal. Thus, the goal about speaking regularly to strangers would need to be discussed in detail-based terms. For example, a person who stammered might have a goal of speaking to strangers and the operational plan would require detailed discussion about how this could be put into practice. It might be the case that the client works in a setting where talking to members of the public might be easy to achieve as a practice task. SFBT advises that a 'doing task' is very important for the first stages in aiming to achieve a goal. The aim is to create new patterns of behaviour. One prompt to use can be seen here: "*to begin reaching your goal, do something that is interesting or fun or unusual. It is important that whatever you decide to do is different from the usual.*"

The aim of getting the client to do something different is that it may facilitate a change in the way the client thinks about the challenges. Staying with the challenge of speaking to strangers, it may be useful to encourage the client to deliberately seek out conversations with strangers in situations where it is unusual for the individual to converse. One client who stammered had reported entering his workplace and turning into the corridor without speaking to the receptionist. Using a SFBT approach the client deliberately made light conversation with the receptionist every time he entered and left the building. His confidence increased following this behaviour.

Specific techniques to use

Scaling has been used in SFBT in order to help set client goals, measure progress and establish priorities for action. It can be used to discover how motivated the client is towards solving the problem and how confident he or she is about doing so. For example, the therapist could ask: *"On a scale of 1-10 how confident are you that you will be able to carry out the telephone call to the travel agent this week?"*

Scaling can be used in an entirely verbal form so that the therapist asks the client to rate themselves or, for clients with speech and language difficulties,

---

Box 6.6 Scaling

In the context of talking to friends in a social setting, the client is asked to rate their experience against the points on the scale. If the client rated him or herself, say, at 2, the therapist might follow this up by exploring with the client what it would take to move to, say 4 (or, perhaps even 2.5). A further use could be to identify where the client wants to get to – is it 10, or would they settle for 8?

10 ... speaking confidently

9

8

7

6

5

4

3

2

1 ... feeling embarrassed about speaking

it may be useful to create a visual display for scaling. This can also be helpful to review progress in a concrete way.

A method which originates from SFBT is the use of the '**miracle question**'. The purpose of this question is to enable the client to think carefully about what would have to happen for a recognizable change to take place. Often the first response from the client may be vague, but the therapist can go on to clarify and check out the client's thinking. 'What else' can frequently be used as a follow-up prompt (O'Connell, 2001). An example of the miracle question is presented below.

> "Suppose one night while you were asleep, there was a miracle and this problem was solved. How would you know? What would be different? Who would be the first person to comment on your change?"
>
> *O'Connell, 2001*

In order to expand and develop the client's thinking about their future, further suggestions for follow-up questions and responses have been suggested (O'Connell, 2001). As with other aspects of this approach it may be necessary for the therapist to help the client understand the question by means of additional linguistic structure and visual signposting. For example, you might find it helpful to explain to the client that you are going to ask what seems like a strange question. It can be a good idea to practise techniques such as the miracle question with a friend or colleague before trying it with a client. The value of a miracle question is that it can be useful in identifying therapy goals as well things that the client is already doing to solve the 'problem' through follow-up questions such as: "*Are there any parts of this miracle happening now? How did you get yourself to do this? What do you suppose needs to happen for this to happen more often?*"

As with all approaches, it is useful for the therapist to develop a repertoire of techniques that can be used at different times with different clients. There are numerous resources on the web that provide specific examples of solution-focused techniques. Often, Solution Focused Brief Therapy courses can be sourced in the UK and further afield. (www.skillsdevelopment.co.uk; www.bps.org.uk). Solution Focused approaches for use with children can be found in material produced by the NSPCC (https://www.nspcc.org.uk/globalassets/documents/publications/solution-focused-practice-toolkit.pdf).

Box 6.7 Miracle question

Practise a miracle question with a friend. Start by asking him or her to think of a problem or issue that they are currently dealing with. The person does not have to tell you what it is. Ask the miracle question and follow it up with prompts to elicit detail.

- What was the first thing you noticed?
- What happened next?
- What did other people notice?
- What else?

Try to elicit a range of responses (thoughts, feelings, and behaviours).

In terms of applicability to the speech and language therapy context, SFBT has been examined with post-stroke aphasic speakers (Northcott, Burns, Simpson, & Hilari, 2015). The study explored the feasibility of solution-focused brief therapy in terms of whether the aphasic speaker could understand the procedures and gain benefit from them. Three men and two women with chronic aphasia took part (age range: 40s–70s) in 3–5 therapy sessions and participants found the therapy acceptable. The study found that it was possible to adapt the approach so that it was accessible to the aphasic speaker. Following the therapy, improvements in mood and communication participation were demonstrated. Measures of social networks, however, remained stable. This small study suggests that solution-focused brief therapy is a promising approach to helping people with aphasia build positive change in their lives. Following on from this, a three-year study aiming to explore how best to adapt the SFBT approach for people with aphasia is at present under way.

Cognitive Behavioural Therapy (CBT)

As described earlier, CBT (see http://www.rcpsych.ac.uk) is based on the principle that emotions are difficult to change directly. It therefore targets distressing emotions by focusing on negative thoughts and behaviours which contribute to the distress. In therapy, the negative thoughts and feelings are challenged with the aim of enabling the client to develop more realistic and adaptive thinking patterns. It has strong empirical support for treating mood and anxiety disorders (Chambless & Ollendick, 2001; DeRubeis & Crits Cristoph, 1998). It has been shown to be successful in treating people with a wide variety of psychological conditions, including anxiety and depression (https://www.rcpsych.ac.uk).

CBT makes use of a number of specific techniques. These might include exposure and graded experiments. For example, a client creates an hierarchy of feared speaking situations and sets a goal of achieving the least fearful, working up to more challenging situations. Predictions of harm (e.g., 'no-one will listen to me') can be tested and new hypotheses can be developed and tested. Cognitive restructuring is another key idea, involving identifying, labelling and challenging unhelpful thoughts.

Thomas et al. (2013) found that behavioural treatments were suitable for people with post-stroke aphasia and low mood. In a randomized controlled trial which evaluated behavioural treatments for this group, 105 people with aphasia were found to have low mood and were randomly split into two groups: one being given behavioural therapies with usual care and the other receiving only usual care. Following 10 sessions the therapy group showed improved self-reported mood, increased self-esteem and observer-related mood.

Behavioural techniques have also been applied to other communication difficulties, including cognitive behavioural therapy used in a range of voice disorders. Butcher, Elias and Cavali (2007) applied a CBT approach to the treatment of psychogenic voice disorders, discussing approaches which take account of the classification of different psychogenic types. In a review of CBT for voice disorders Miller et al. (2014) demonstrated positive outcomes for

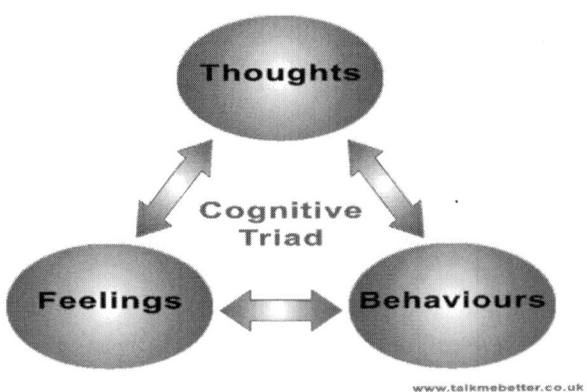

Figure 6.1 Framework for CBT.

voice therapy which includes CBT. People with Aspergers Syndrome may also benefit from this approach (Attwood, 2004). A number of studies have found that CBT, delivered either face-to-face or online, can be effective in reducing social anxiety for adults who stammer (e.g., Helgadóttir, Menzies, Onslow, Packman, & O'Brian, 2009; Menzies et al., 2008). Menzies, Onslow, Packman, and O'Brian (2009) published a tutorial for speech and language therapists on adapting CBT for working with speech-related anxiety in adults who stammer which also includes a helpful summary of CBT principles.

Narrative Therapy

Narrative Therapy was developed in the 1970s and 1980s by Michael White and David Epston in Australia and New Zealand (Epston & White, 1990). It is intended to be a nonjudgemental approach which centres people as experts in their own lives. Problems are viewed as separate from individuals and it assumes that individuals have skills, competencies and beliefs which will enable them to change the difficult situation in their lives. The individual (or a group of people) will talk about their difficulty using the framework of a 'story' which may be dominant or alternative. The events in the individual's story will be linked together through discussion with the therapist and used to develop future actions aiming to bring about change. Wolter, Di Lollo and Apel (2006) describe a narrative approach to counselling for use with adolescents and adults with language-literacy difficulties. This approach is shown to be useful with a 22-year-old student who is receiving literacy intervention and has low self-esteem. Three main phases are described in this approach. Firstly, the therapist encourages the client to externalize the problem, suggesting they talk about it in the third person. Secondly, the therapist helps the client to map the influence of the problem on their life ensuring there is a deep, full and detailed description. Finally, the individual talks about the influence of the person on the life of the problem, responding to a set of specified questions from the therapist. In this paper, the student reports changes following therapy, finding viable solutions and developing an alternative self-narrative. In a more specific application to the speech and language therapy context DiLollo, Neimeyer and Manning (2002) report the use of narrative therapy to respond to a relapse in stuttering speech. Here, the client is given narrative therapy to enhance the construct of fluent speech and the meaningfulness of the fluent speaker role. Clearly, from these papers it can be seen that there are some opportunities to develop the role of narrative therapy further in speech and language therapy settings.

Mindfulness

Mindfulness has come into prominence recently and has been applied to both clinical and non-clinical populations. Descriptions of how to 'do it' can be seen in self-help books, magazine articles and Apps as well as academic journals. It can be described as present moment awareness where the individual learns to concentrate on the unfolding present moment whatever the experience. A well-known and relatively simple explanation of mindfulness is that provided by Kabat-Zinn (1994) where it is cited as "paying attention in a particular way: on purpose, in the present moment, and non-judgementally" (p.4). There has been academic discussion about the definition of mindfulness with a well-accepted definition emerging from work by Bishop, Lau et al. (2004). These authors propose a two-component model of mindfulness, using testable evidence to describe this model.

> **Component 1**: Self-regulation of attention so that it is maintained on the individual's immediate experience, thereby allowing for increased recognition of mental events in the present moment.

> **Component 2**: Adopting a particular orientation toward one's experiences in the present moment, an orientation that is characterized by curiosity, openness, and acceptance.

In these two components, it would be possible for the client to increase their awareness of anxiety and negative thoughts about speaking. This is highlighted by Boyle (2011) in relation to stammering. The aim of increasing focus and exposure to a feared issue may cause the feeling to reduce or be extinguished. Authors note that the client is not required to use a specific technique, such as relaxation, but to just notice their thoughts which arise in their stream of consciousness.

There is some evidence to suggest that mindfulness meditation can improve attention in neurologically-intact individuals and, subsequently, some research has been reported where this approach has been used with people with aphasia. The research question has focused around the issue of whether mindfulness can enhance the individual's attention as, following stroke or other neurological disease, there is evidence to show that the brain cannot allocate resources sufficiently well to various cognitive processes. Laures-Gore and Marshall (2016) reported a single case where an adult with aphasia was trained with the mindfulness technique with pre- and post-assessments being given for comparison. The assessments included measures of language, attention and physiological measures of cortisol and heart rate variability. These were undertaken as two baseline measures followed by immediate post training and then one-week post training. Changes were found in the physiological and behavioural measures, including word productivity, phrase length, word generation and increased attention. Another study (Orenstein, Basilakos, & Marshall, 2012) examined three individuals with aphasia following mindfulness training, and although no improvements in language were demonstrated there was some evidence for increased reaction time. There has also been some interest (and useful summaries of techniques), though little in the way of research, to using mindfulness training and the related approach of acceptance and commitment therapy when working with people who stammer (Beilby & Byrnes, 2012; Boyle, 2011) .

Personal supervision

All therapists need to be able to respond appropriately to whatever the patient talks about, and for speech and language therapists there may be patients who describe very distressing experiences. If this happens then the therapist can find challenges in knowing what to say and what to do. Often those patients are the ones which create anxiety and uncertainty for the therapist, who may reflect on their own response and worry about whether it was appropriate and helpful (and see also the discussion on emotional labour and 'burnout' in Chapter 3). This is where personal supervision may be relevant, not only for newly-qualified therapists but also for those who have longer experience but who may be challenged by patients with complex emotional circumstances. Supervision can give the therapist feedback on their reported behaviours and thoughts which can enable them to develop useful viewpoints for moving forward with a client. An additional benefit is that it can provide a secure base to explore therapeutic approaches.

Managerial and professional supervision is required in health service provision and can enable the therapist to develop useful viewpoints for enhancing professional skills (see HCPC Standards of Proficiency, 2014). However, there is less formal awareness about the personal impact on the therapist and how this can be managed. This may focus on therapists who need to discuss their feelings about the challenging situations they confront and develop further personal capacities to cope with the issues raised by patients in the clinical setting. Subsequently, various services have created supervision opportunities which may come under the title of mentoring or be found in group multiprofessional supervisory settings. In an early paper, Green (1995) reported on the level of stress experienced by speech and language therapists and the need for enhanced supervision and understanding of what counselling means.

Parkinson and Rae (1996) examined four groups (first- and fourth-year students, new and experienced therapists, total 151) who completed a questionnaire exploring counselling behaviours used by therapists and students. In addition, the groups were asked to report teaching work behaviours. First-year students indicated fewer counselling behaviours than fourth-year students and experienced therapists. Fourth-year students anticipated using less teaching behaviour than was reported by new and experienced therapists. The authors discussed the role of further training in counselling and the personal therapy which may be relevant for current understanding. Syder and Levy (1998) discuss the role of and need for personal supervision in a useful chapter. The RCSLT have developed a wide range of information and resources for speech and language supervision, available as part of CQ Live from their webpages: (https://www.rcslt.org/cq_live/resources_a_z/supervision/supervision).

Conclusions

There is no single psychological model which relates entirely to the practice of speech and language therapy and explains the process of helping and enabling the communicatively-impaired client to respond, cope and improve their wellbeing. Speech and language therapy has been required to extrapolate material from psychological literature and apply it to the communication difficulties context. Many of the approaches and models outlined here contain overlapping principles and techniques, albeit they are described using different language. For example, 'narratives' and 'personal constructs' seem to have much in common and the concept of 'externalising the problem' in narrative therapy and 'identifying and labelling unhelpful thoughts' in CBT perform similar functions. The important idea for the speech and language therapist to take away is the value in developing a range of techniques that can support clients to make changes and to do this in the context of providing an accepting and empathetic therapy environment where clients have opportunity to express anxieties, sadness or, maybe, even joy. Finally, whilst there is some evidence that counselling approaches in speech and language therapy have been of benefit, the research and academic literature still needs to develop further, a comment that has been echoed throughout the chapters in this book.

Box 6.8 Qualities

What qualities would you choose in someone you wanted to discuss a problem with? Who wouldn't you choose?

Try and identify some characteristics which would make you unlikely to talk openly with someone.

References

The Autistic Society. (2013). *Ageing with Autism – A Handbook for Care and Support Professionals*. Godalming, UK: The Autistic Society.

Al Anbar, N.N., Dardennes, R.M., Prado-Netto, A., Kaye, K., & Contejean, Y. (2010). Treatment choices in autism spectrum disorder: The role of parental illness perceptions. *Research in Developmental Disabilities, 31*(3), 817–828.

Alzheimer's Society. https://www.alzheimers.org.uk/download/downloads/id/1768/factsheet_depression_and_anxiety.pdf

Alzheimer's Society. https://www.alzheimers.org.uk/info/20046/help_with_dementia_care/31/understanding_and_supporting_a_person_with_dementia/4

Alzheimer's Society. https://www.alzheimers.org.uk/download/downloads/id/1766/factsheet_what_is_young-onset_dementia.pdf

American Psychological Association (2010). *Resilience and Recovery after War: Refugee Children and Families in the US*. Washington, D.C. http://www.apa.org/pi/families/refugess.aspx

Anderson, G. (1997) Post stroke depression and pathological crying: Clinical aspects and new pharmacological approaches. *Aphasiology, 11*, 651–664.

Armstrong, M.J. (2017). Shared decision-making in stroke: An evolving approach to improved patient care. *Stroke and Vascular Neurology, (2)*3. Doi: 10.1136/svn-2017-000081

Attwood, T. (2004). CBT for children and adolescents with asperger's syndrome. *Behaviour Change, 21*(3), 147-161.

https://www.autism.com/understanding_advice

Autistic Society (http://autism.org.uk)

Autistica (http://autistica.org.uk)

Badolamenti, S., Sili, A., Caruso, R., & Fida, R. (2017). What do we know about emotional labour in nursing? A narrative review. *British Journal of Nursing, 26*(1), 48–55.

Baggs, T.W. (2013). Has speech-language pathology changed? Personality types of contemporary students. *The Internet Journal of Allied Health Sciences and Practice, 11*. Retrieved from http://nsuworks.nova.edu/cgi/viewcontent.cgi?article=1427&context=ijahsp

Baker, E. (2010). The experience of discharging children from phonological intervention. *International Journal of Speech-Language Pathology, 12*(4), 325–328.

Balint, M. (1964). *The Doctor, His Patient and the Illness*. London: Pitman Medical.

Bandura, A. (1995). *Self Efficacy in Changing Societies*. New York: Cambridge University Press.

Bandura, A. (1977). Self-efficacy: Toward a unifying theory of behaviour change. *Psychological Review, 84*, 191–215.

Bandura, A. (2000). Health promotion from the perspective of social cognitive theory. In P. Norman, C. Abraham, & M. Conner (Eds), *Understanding and Changing Health Behaviour* (pp.299–339). Reading, UK: Harwood.

Barton, J. (2009). Interdisciplinary approaches to the assessment and management of well-being. In: S.M. Brumfitt (Ed.), *Psychological Well-being and Acquired Communication Impairments*. Chichester: Wiley-Blackwell.

Baxter, S., Johnson, M., Blank, L., Cantrell, A., Brumfitt, S., Enderby, P., & Goyder, E. (2015). The state of the art in non-pharmacological interventions for developmental stuttering. Part 1: A systematic review of effectiveness. *International Journal of Language & Communication Disorders, 50*(5), 676–718. https://doi.org/10.1111/1460-6984.12171

Beck, A.T. (1970). Cognitive therapy: Nature and relation to behavior therapy. *Behavior Therapy, 1*, 184–200.

Beilby, J.M. & Byrnes, M.L. (2012). Acceptance and commitment therapy for people who stutter. *Perspectives on Fluency & Fluency Disorders, 22*(1), 34–46.

Bekker, H. (2014). Designing decision aids that work in practice. Paper presented at the RCSLT Mind the Gap: Putting Research into Practice conference, Leeds.

Bellarosa, C. & Chen, P.Y. (1997). The effectiveness and practicality of occupational stress management interventions: A survey of subject matter expert opinions. *Journal of Occupational Health Psychology, 2*, 247–262.

Bellon-Harn, M.L. & Garrett, M.T. (2008). VISION: A model of cultural responsiveness for speech-language pathologists working in family partnerships. *Communication Disorders Quarterly, 29*(3), 141–148.

Besley, J., Kayes, N.M., & McPherson, K.M. (2011). Assessing therapeutic relationships in physiotherapy: Literature review. *New Zealand Journal of Physiotherapy, 39*(2), 81–91.

Bishop, S.R., Lau, M., Shapiro, S., Carlson, L., Anderson, N.,...Devins, G. (2004). Mindfulness: A proposed operational definition. *Clinical Psychology Science and Practice, 11*(3), 230–241.

Bogart, K.R. (2014) The role of disability self concept in adaptation to congenital or acquired disability. *Rehabilitation Psychology, 59*(1), 107–115.

Bolton, S.C. (2000). Who cares? Offering emotion work as a "gift" in the nursing labour process. *Journal of Advanced Nursing, 32*(3), 580–586.

Bonanno, G.A. (2008). Loss, trauma, and human resilience: Have we underestimated the human capacity to thrive after extremely aversive events? *Psychological Trauma: Theory, Research, Practice, and Policy, S*(1), 101–113. https://doi.org/10.1037/1942-9681.S.1.101

Bond, T. (1993) *Standards and Ethics for Counselling in Action*. London: Sage.

Bonsaksen, T. (2013). Self-reported therapeutic style in occupational therapy students. *The British Journal of Occupational Therapy, 76*(11), 496–502.

Bordin, E.S. (1979). The generalizability of the psychoanalytic concept of the working alliance. *Psychotherapy: Theory, Research & Practice, 16*(3), 252–260.

Botheridge, C.M. & Grandey A.A. (2002). Emotional labor and burnout: Comparing two perspectives of "people work". *Journal of Vocational Behaviour, 60*(1), 17–39.

Bowling, A. & Dieppe, P. (2005). What is successful ageing and who should define it? *BMJ, 331*, 1548-1551.

Boyle, M.P. (2011). Mindfulness training in stuttering therapy: A tutorial for speech-language pathologists. *Journal of Fluency Disorders, 36*(2), 122-129.

Bright, F.A.S., Kayes, N.M., McCann, C.M., & McPherson, K.M. (2013). Hope in people with aphasia. *Aphasiology, 27*(1), 41-58.

Brissette, I., Scheier, M.F., & Carver, C.S. (2002). The role of optimism in social network development, coping, and psychological adjustment during a life transition. *Journal of Personality and Social Psychology, 82*(1), 102-111.

Broadbent, E., Ellis, C.J., Thomas, J., Gamble, G., & Petrie, K.J. (2009). Can an illness perception intervention reduce illness anxiety in spouses of myocardial infarction patients? A randomized controlled trial. *Journal of Psychosomatic Research, 67*(1), 11-15.

Bromley, D. (1974). *The Psychology of Human Ageing.* London: Pelican.

Brown, D. & Knox, M. (2010). Group therapy: An interprofessional approach. In S.M. Brumfitt (Ed.) *Psychological Well-Being and Acquired Communication Impairments,* (pp.175-197). Chichester: Wiley-Blackwell.

Brown, M.A., McIntyre, L.L., Crnic, K.A., Baker, B.L., & Blacher, J. (2011). Preschool children with and without developmental delay: Risk, parenting, and child demandingness. *Journal of Mental Health Research in Intellectual Disabilities, 4*, 206-226.

Bronfenbrenner, U. (1979) *The Ecology of Human Development: Experiments by Nature and Design.* Cambridge, MA: Harvard University Press.

Broom, A. (2005). Virtually He@lthy: The impact of internet use on disease experience and the doctor–patient relationship. *Qualitative Health Research, 15*(3), 325-345.

Brumfitt, S.M. (1985). The use of repertory grids with aphasic people. In N. Beail (Ed.) *Repertory Grid Technique and Personal Constructs.* London: Croom Helm.

Brumfitt, S.M. (1993). Losing your sense of self: What aphasia can do. *Aphasiology, 7*(6), 569-575.

Brumfitt, S.M. (1998). The measurement of psychological well being in the person with a communication disorder. *International Journal of Language and Communication Science, 33*, 116-121.

Brumfitt, S.M. (2006). Psychosocial aspects of aphasia: Speech and language therapists' views on professional practice. *Disability and Rehabilitation, April 28*(8), 523-534.

Brumfitt S.M. & Sheeran, P. (1999). The development and validation of the Visual Analogue Self-esteem Scale (VASES). *British Journal of Clinical Psychology, 38*, 387-400.

Brumfitt, S. & Sheeran, P. (2010). *VASES: Visual Analogue Self-Esteem Scale, 1st ed.* Milton Keynes: Routledge.

Buck, F., Drinnan, M., Wilson, J., & Barnard, I.S. (2007). What are the illness perceptions of people with dysphonia: A pilot study. *The Journal of Laryngology and Otology, 121*(1), 31-39.

Buetow, S., Jutel, A., & Hoare, K. (2009). Shrinking social space in the doctor–modern patient relationship: A review of forces for, and implications of, homologisation. *Patient Education and Counseling*, 74(1), 97–103.

Burns, K. (2005). *Focus on Solutions*. London: Whurr.

Burns, K. (2010) Solution Focused Brief Therapy for people with acquired communication impairments. In: S.M. Brumfitt (Ed.), *Psychological Well-being and Acquired Communication Impairments*. Chichester UK: Wiley-Blackwell.

Bury, M. (1991). The sociology of chronic illness: A review of research and prospects. *Sociology of Health and Illness*, 13, 451–468.

Butcher, P., Elias, A., & Cavalli, L. (2007). *Understanding and Treating Psychogenic Voice Disorder: A CBT Framework*. Chichester: John Wiley & Sons.

Bylund, C.L., Gueguen, J.A., Sabee, C.M., Imes, R.S., Li, Y., & Sanford, A.A. (2007). Provider–patient dialogue about internet health information: An exploration of strategies to improve the provider–patient relationship. *Patient Education and Counseling*, 66(3), 346–352.

Byng, S., Cairns, D., & Duchan, J. (2002). Values in practice and practising values. *Journal of Communication Disorders*, 35(2), 89–106.

Cameron, L.D. & Leventhal, H. (2003). *The Self-regulation of Health and Illness Behaviour*. Hove: Psychology Press.

Carey, B., O'Brian, S., Lowe, R., & Onslow, M. (2014). Webcam delivery of the Camperdown Program for adolescents who stutter: A phase II trial. *Language, Speech, and Hearing Services in Schools*, 45(4), 314–324.

Carroll, C. (2010). "It's not every day that parents get a chance to talk like this": Exploring parents' perceptions and expectations of speech-language pathology services for children with intellectual disability. *International Journal of Speech-Language Pathology*, 12(4), 352–361.

Carver, C.S. (1997). You want to measure coping but your protocol's too long: Consider the Brief COPE. *International Journal of Behavioral Medicine*, 4, 92–100.

Chadwick, D.D., Jolliffe, J., Goldbart, J., & Burton, M.H. (2006). Barriers to caregiver compliance with eating and drinking recommendations for adults with intellectual disabilities and dysphagia. *Journal of Applied Research in Intellectual Disabilities*, 19(2), 153–162. https://doi.org/10.1111/j.1468-3148.2005.00250.x

Chambless, D.L. & Ollendick, T.H. (2001) Empirically supported psychological interventions: Controversies and evidence. *Annual Review of Psychology*, 52, 685–716.

Charmaz, L. (2002). The self as habit: The reconstruction of self in chronic illness. *Occupation Participation and Health*, 22 Supp 1, 31S–41S.

Childrens and Families Act (2014) http://www.legislation.gov.uk

Chopik, W. (2017). Associations among relational values, support, health, and well-being across the adult lifespan. *Personal Relationships*, 24, 408–422.

Clegg, J., Hollis, C., Mawhood, L., & Rutter, M. (2005). Developmental language disorders: A follow up in later life adult life. Cognitive, language and psychosocial outcomes. *Child Psychology and Psychiatry*, 46(2), 128–149.

Collins, C. & Rochfort, A. (2016). Promoting self-management and patient empowerment in primary care. In O. Capelli (Ed.), *Primary Care in Practice – Integration is Needed* (Ch. 2). InTech, doi: 10.5772/62763. Available from: https://www.intechopen.com/books/primary-care-in-practice-integration-is-needed/promoting-self-management-and-patient-empowerment-in-primary-care

Colodny, N. (2005). Dysphagic independent feeders' justifications for noncompliance with recommendations by a speech-language pathologist. *American Journal of Speech Language Pathology, 14,* 61-70.

Coltart, N. (1993). *How to Survive as a Psychotherapist.* London: Sheldon Press.

Connell, J., Grant, S., & Mullin, T. (2006). Client initiated termination of therapy at NHS primary care counselling services. *Counsel Psychother Res, 6,* 60–67.

Conner, M. & Norman, P. (Eds). (1996*). Predicting Health Behaviour: Research and Practice with Social Cognition Models.* Buckingham: Open University Press.

http://counsellingtutor.com/counselling-approaches/person-centred-approach-to-counselling/carl-rogers-core-conditions/

Cribb, A. (2011). Involvement, shared decision-making and medicines. London: Royal Pharmaceutical Society. Retrieved from: http://www.rpharms.com/

Crichton-Smith, I. (2002). Communicating in the real world: Accounts from people who stammer. *Journal of Fluency Disorders, 27*(4), 333–352.

Cruice, M., Worrall, L., Hickson, L., & Murison, R. (2009). Measuring quality of life: Comparing family members' and friends' ratings with those of their aphasic partners. *Aphasiology, 19,* 111–129.

Cumming, E. & Henry, W. (1961). *Growing Old: The Process of Disengagement.* New York: Basic Books.

Dalton, P. (1994). *Counselling People with Communication Problems.* London: Sage.

Darley, F.L. (1975). Treatment of acquired aphasia. In W.J. Friedlander (Ed.), *Advances in Neurology,* Vol 7. New York: Raven Press.

Darviri, C., Demakakos, P., Tigani, X., Charizani, F., Tsiou, C., Tsagkari, C., Monos, D. (2009). Psychosocial dimensions of exceptional longevity: A qualitative exploration of centenarians' experiences, personality, and life strategies. *Aging and Human Development, 69*(2), 101-118.

Davidson, K. (2002). The sociology of later life. In P. Woodrow (Ed), *Ageing: Issues for Physical, Psychological and Social Health.* London: Whurr.

DeRubeis, R.J. & Crits-Cristoph, P. (1998). Empirically supported individual and group psychological treatments for adult mental disorders. *Consulting Clinical Psychology, 66*(1), 37-52.

de Sonneville-Koedoot, C., Bouwmans, C., Franken, M.-C., & Stolk, E. (2015). Economic evaluation of stuttering treatment in preschool children: The RESTART-study. *Journal of Communication Disorders, 58,* 106–118.

Dedding, C., van Doorn, R., Winkler, L., & Reis, R. (2011). How will e-health affect patient participation in the clinic? A review of e-health studies and the current evidence for changes in the relationship between medical professionals and patients. *Social Science & Medicine*, *72*(1), 49–53.

DiLollo, A. & Favreau, C. (2010). Person-centered care and Speech and Language Therapy. *Seminars in Speech and Language*, *31*(02), 90–97.

DiLollo, A., Neimeyer, R.A., & Manning, W.H. (2002). A personal construct psychology view of relapse: Indications for a narrative therapy component to stuttering treatment. *Journal of Fluency Disorders*, *27*, 19–42.

DiMatteo, M.R & Di Nicola, D.D. (1982). *Achieving Patient Compliance: The Psychology of the Medical Practitioner's Role*. New York: Pergamon.

DuBay, M.F., Laures-Gore, J.S., Matheny, K., & Romski, M.A. (2011). Coping resources in individuals with aphasia. *Aphasiology*, *25*(9), 1016–1029. https://doi.org/10.1080/0 2687038.2011.570933

Ebert, K.D. (2017). Measuring clinician–client relationships in speech-language treatment for school-age children. *American Journal of Speech-Language Pathology*, *26*(1), 146–152.

Ebert, K.D. & Kohnert, K. (2010). Common factors in speech-language treatment: An exploratory study of effective clinicians. *Journal of Communication Disorders*, *43*(2), 133–147.

Egan, G. (2009). *The Skilled Helper: A Problem-Management and Opportunity-Development Approach to Helping*. Boston, MA: Cengage Learning.

ELSA English Longitudinal Study of Ageing. http://www.ifs.org.uk/elsa

El Sharkawi, A., Ramig, L., Logemann, J.A., Pauloski, B.R., Rademaker, A.W., Smith, C.H., … Werner, C. (2002). Swallowing and voice effects of Lee Silverman Voice Treatment (LSVT): A pilot study. *Journal of Neurology, Neurosurgery, and Psychiatry*, *72*(1), 31–36.

Emanuel, J. & Emanuel, L. (1992). Four models of the physician–patient relationship. *JAMA*, *267*(16), 2221–2226.

Enderby, P. & John, A. (2015). *Therapy Outcome Measures for Rehabilitation Professionals*, *3rd ed.* Guildford: J&R Press Ltd.

Epston, D. & White, M. (1990). *Narrative Means to Therapeutic Ends*. New York: Norton.

Equalities Act (2010). http://www. legislation.gov.uk

Erickson, S. & Block, S. (2013). The social and communicative impact of stuttering on adolescents and their families. *Journal of Fluency Disorders*, *38*(4), 311–324.

Erikson, E.H. (1968). *Identity: Youth and Crisis*. New York: W.W. Norton.

Eysenck, H.J. & Eysenck, M.W. (1985). *Personality and Individual Differences: A Natural Science Approach*. New York: Plenum.

Ferguson, A. & Armstrong, E. (2004). Reflections on speech-language therapists' talk: Implications for clinical practice and education. *International Journal of Language & Communication Disorders*, *39*(4), 469–477.

Ferguson, M. & Spence, W. (2012). Towards a definition: What does "health promotion" mean to speech and language therapists? *International Journal of Language & Communication Disorders, 47*(5), 522–533.

Floyd, J., Zebrowski, P.M., & Flamme, G.A. (2007). Stages of change and stuttering: A preliminary view. *Journal of Fluency Disorders, 32*(2), 95–120.

Forsingdal, S., St John, W., Harvey, A., & Wearne, P. (2013). Goal setting with mothers in child development services. *Child: Care, Health and Development, 30*, 265–296.

Fourie, R., Crowley, N., & Oliviera, A. (2011). A qualitative exploration of therapeutic relationships from the perspective of six children receiving speech-language therapy. *Topics in Language Disorders, 31*(4), 310–324.

Fourie, R.J. (2009). Qualitative study of the therapeutic relationship in speech and language therapy: Perspectives of adults with acquired communication and swallowing disorders. *International Journal of Language & Communication Disorders, 44*(6), 979–999.

Foxwell, R., Morley, C., & Frizelle, D. (2013). Illness perceptions, mood and quality of life: A systematic review of coronary heart disease patients. *Journal of Psychosomatic Research, 75*(3), 211–222.

Fransella, F. (1972). *Personal Change and Reconstruction.* New York: Academic Press.

Fratiglioni, L., Paillard-Borg, S., & Winblad, B. (2004). An active and socially integrated lifestyle in late life might protect against dementia. *THE LANCET Neurology, 3.* http://neurology.thelancet.com

Fredrickson, B.L. (2001). The role of positive emotions in positive psychology. *The American Psychologist, 56*(3), 218–226.

Fredrickson, B.L. & Losada, M.F. (2005). Positive affect and the complex dynamics of human flourishing. *American Psychologist, 60*(7), 678–686.

Freshwater, D. (2004). Emotional intelligence: Developing emotional literate training in mental health. *Mental Health Practice, 8*, 12–15.

Freud, S. (1933). *New Introductory Lectures on Psycho-Analysis.* The Standard Edition of the Complete Psychological Works of Sigmund Freud, Volume XXII (1932-1936).

Fromm, D., Holland, A., Armstrong, E., Forbes, M., MacWhinney, B., Risko, A., & Mattison, N. (2011). "Better but no cigar": Persons with aphasia speak about their speech. *Aphasiology, 25*(11), 1431–1447.

Fuller, A. (2010). Speech and language therapy in Sure Start Local Programmes: A survey-based analysis of practice and innovation. *International Journal of Language & Communication Disorders, 45*(2), 182–203.

Geldard, K., Geldard, D., & Yin Foo, R. (2013). *Counselling Children: A Practical Introduction, 3rd ed.* London: Sage.

Geller, E. & Foley, G.M. (2009). Expanding the "ports of entry" for speech-language pathologists: A relational and reflective model for clinical practice. *American Journal of Speech-Language Pathology, 18*(1), 4–21.

Gerber, B.S. & Eiser, A.R. (2001). The patient-physician relationship in the Internet age: Future prospects and the research agenda. *Journal of Medical Internet Research, 3*(2), 5.

Glidden, L.M. & Natcher, A.L. (2009). Coping strategy use, personality, and adjustment of parents rearing children with developmental disabilities. *Journal of Intellectual Disability Research, 53*(12), 998–1013.

Glogowska, M. & Campbell, R. (2000). Investigating parental views of involvement in pre-school speech and language therapy. *International Journal of Language & Communication Disorders, 35*(3), 391–405.

Gollwitzer, P.M. (1999). Implementation intentions: Strong effects of simple plans. *American Psychologist, 54*, 493–503.

Grandey, A.A. (2000). Emotion regulation in the workplace: A new way to conceptualize emotional labor. *Journal of Occupational Health Psychology, 5*(1), 95–110.

Grandey, A., Foo, S.C., Groth, M., & Goodwin, R.E. (2012). Free to be you and me: A climate of authenticity alleviates burnout from emotional labor. *Journal of Occupational Health Psychology, 17*(1), 1–14.

Gravell, R. (1988). *Communication Problems in Elderly People: Practical Approaches to Management.* London: Croom Helm.

Green, R. (1995). Non managerial supervision as a statutory requirement for the SLT profession. *International Journal of Language and Communication Disorders, 30*(51), 551–558.

Grencavage, L.M. & Norcross, J.C. (1990). Where are the commonalities among the therapeutic common factors? *Professional Psychology: Research and Practice, 21*(5), 372–378.

Gum, A., Snyder, C.R., & Duncan, P.W. (2006). Hopeful thinking, participation, and depressive symptoms three months after stroke. *Psychology & Health, 21*(3), 319–334.

Hagger, M.S. & Orbell, S. (2003). A meta-analytic review of the common-sense model of illness representations. *Psychology and Health, 18(2)*, 141-184.

Havighurst, R. (1963). Successful ageing. In R. Williams, C. Tibbetts, & W. Donahoe (Eds), *Processes of Aging*, pp.311-315. Chicago: University of Chicago Press.

Hawley, S.T. & Morris, A.M. (2017). Cultural challenges to engaging patients in shared decision making. *Patient Education and Counseling, 100*(1), 18–24.

Health Care and Professions Council (2014). Standards of Proficiency. London: Health Care and Professions Council.

Helgadóttir, F.D., Menzies, R.G., Onslow, M., Packman, A., & O'Brian, S. (2009). Online CBT II: A phase I trial of a standalone, online CBT treatment program for social anxiety in stuttering. *Behaviour Change, 26*(4), 254–270.

Hendry, L.B. & Kloep, M. (2002) *Lifespan Development: Resources, Challenges and Risks.* London: Thomson Learning. https://www.cengage.co.uk/education/

Herbert, R., Haw, C., Brown, C., Gregory, E., & Brumfitt, S. (2012). *Accessible Information Guidelines.* The Stroke Association.

Hersh, D. (2001). Experiences of ending aphasia therapy. *International Journal of Language & Communication Disorders, 36 Suppl*, 80–85.

Hersh, D. (2003). "Weaning" clients from aphasia therapy: Speech pathologists' strategies for discharge. *Aphasiology, 17*(11), 1007–1029.

Hersh, D. (2010). "I can't sleep at night with discharging this lady": The personal impact of ending therapy on speech-language pathologists. *International Journal of Speech-Language Pathology, 12*(4), 283–291.

Heyduck, K., Meffert, C., & Glattacker, M. (2014). Illness and treatment perceptions of patients with chronic low back pain: Characteristics and relation to individual, disease and interaction variables. *Journal of Clinical Psychology in Medical Settings, 21*(3), 267–281.

Hibbard, J. & Gilburt, H. (2014). *Supporting People to Manage their Health. An Introduction to Patient Activation*. London: The Kings Fund.

Hibbard, J.H. & Green, J. (2011). "Who are we reaching through the patient portal?": Engaging the already engaged. *The International Journal of Person Centered Medicine, 1*(4), 788–793.

Hibbard, J.H., Mahoney, E.R., Stockard, J., & Tusler, M. (2005). Development and testing of a short form of the Patient Activation Measure. *Health Services Research, 40*(6 Pt 1), 1918–1930.

Hilari, K., Northcott, S., Roy, P., Marshall, J., Wiggins, R.D., Chataway, J., & Ames, D. (2010). Psychological distress after stroke and aphasia: The first six months. *Clinical Rehabilitation, 24*(2), 181–190.

Hochschild, A. (1983). *The Managed Heart: Commercialization of Human Feeling*. Berkeley, CA: University of California Press.

Hoffman, T. & Worrall, L. (2004). Designing effective written health education materials: Considerations for health professionals. *Disability and Rehabilitation,* 26, 1166–1173.

Holland, A. (2007) *Counseling in Communication Disorders, 2nd ed.* San Diego: Plural Publishing.

Holland, A. & Nelson, R. (2014). *Counselling in Communication Disorders. A Wellbeing Perspective, 2nd ed.* San Diego, CA: Plural Publishing.

Holmes, T.H. & Rahe, R.H. (1967). The Social Readjustment Rating Scale. *Journal of Psychosomatic Research, 11*(2), 213–218.

Horne, R. (2001). Compliance, adherence and concordance. In K. Taylor & G. Harding (Eds). *Pharmacy Practice*. London: Taylor & Francis.

Horne, R. & Weinman, J. (2002). Self-regulation and self-management in asthma: Exploring the role of illness perceptions and treatment beliefs in explaining non-adherence to preventer medication. *Psychology and Health, 17*(1), 17–32.

Hoy, R. (2006). Autism and me. http://www.roryhoy.com/autism-me

Hutnik, N., Smith, P., & Koch, T. (2012). What does it feel like to be 100? Socio emotional aspects of well being in the stories of 16 centenarians living in the UK. *Ageing and Mental Health, 16*(7), 811–818.

ICAN. Factsheet A. http://www.ican.org.uk

Illness Perceptions Questionnaire (PPQ). http://www.uib.no/ipq/

James, N. (1989). Emotional labour: Skill and work in the social regulation of feelings. *Sociological Review, 37*, 15-42.

Joffe, V., Beverley, A., & Scott, L. (2011). My speech, language and communication: "A real kind of overwhelming kind of challenge sometime". In K. Hilari & N. Botting (Eds),*The Impact of Communication Disability across the Lifespan.* Sussex: J&R Press.

Johnson, F.M., Best, W., Beckley, F.C., Maxim, J., & Beeke, S. (2016). Identifying mechanisms of change in a conversation therapy for aphasia using behaviour change theory and qualitative methods. *International Journal of Language & Communication Disorders, 52*(3), 374-387.

Johnson, M. & Elias, A. (2010). *East Kent Outcome System, Revised Editions.* East Kent: East Kent Coastal Primary Care Trust.

Johnston, D.W. (1989). Will stress management prevent coronary heart disease? *The Psychologist: Bulletin of the British Psychological Society, 7*, 275-278.

Kaba, R. & Sooriakumaran, P. (2007). The evolution of the doctor-patient relationship. *International Journal of Surgery, 5*(1), 57-65.

Kabat-Zinn, J. (1994). *Wherever You Go, There You Are: Mindfulness Meditation in Everyday Life.* New York: Hyperion.

Kahneman, D. (2011). *Thinking, Fast and Slow.* New York: Farrar, Straus and Giroux.

Kanner, A.D., Coyne, J.C., Schaefer, C., & Lazarus, R.S. (1981). Comparison of two modes of stress measurement: Daily hassles and uplifts versus major life events. *Journal of Behavioral Medicine, 4*(1), 1-39.

Kaptchuk, T.J., Kelley, J.M., Conboy, L.A., Davis, R.B., Kerr, C.E., Jacobson, E.E., ... Lembo, A.J. (2008). Components of placebo effect: Randomised controlled trial in patients with irritable bowel syndrome. *BMJ, 336*(7651), 999-1003.

Kelchner, L. (2013). Telehealth and the treatment of voice disorders: A discussion regarding evidence. *Perspectives on Voice & Voice Disorders, 23*(3), 88-94.

Kelly, G. (1955). *The Psychology of Personal Constructs.* New York: W.W. Norton.

Kendall, E., Catalano, T., Kuipers, P., Posner, N., Buys, N., & Charker, J. (2007). Recovery following stroke: The role of self-management education. *Social Science & Medicine, 64*(3), 735-746.

Kitson, A., Marshall, A., Bassett, K., & Zeitz, K. (2013). What are the core elements of patient-centred care? A narrative review and synthesis of the literature from health policy, medicine and nursing. *Journal of Advanced Nursing, 69*(1), 4-15.

Kloep, M., Hendry, L.B., & Saunders, D. (2009). A new perspective on human development. *Conference of the International Journal of Arts and Sciences, 1*(6), 332-343.

Lai, W.W., Goh, T.J., Oei, T.P.S., & Sung, M. (2015). Coping and well-being in parents of children with autism spectrum disorders (ASD). *Journal of Autism and Developmental Disorders, 45*(8), 2582-2593.

Lambert, M.J. (1992). Psychotherapy outcome research: Implications for integrative and eclectic therapists. In J.C. Norcross & M.R. Goldfried (Eds), *Handbook of Psychotherapy Integration*. New York: Basic Books.

Lambert, M.J. & Bergin, A.E. (1994). The effectiveness of psychotherapy. In A.E. Bergin & S.L. Garfield (Eds), *Handbook of Psychotherapy and Behavior Change, 4th ed.* New York: John Wiley & Sons Ltd.

Lambert, M.J. & Ogles, B.M. (2004). The efficacy and effectiveness of psychotherapy. In M.J. Lambert (Ed.), *Bergin and Garfield's Handbook of Psychotherapy and Behaviour Change*, 5th ed. pp.139-193. New York: Wiley.

Laska, K.M., Gurman, A.S., & Wampold, B.E. (2014). Expanding the lens of evidence-based practice in psychotherapy: A common factors perspective. *Psychotherapy, 51*(4), 467–481. https://doi.org/10.1037/a0034332

Laures-Gore, J. & Marshall, R.S. (2016). Mindfulness meditation in aphasia: A case report. *Neurorehabilitation, 38*(4), 321-329.

Law, J., Reilly, S., & Snow, P.C. (2013). Child speech, language and communication needs re-examined in a public health context: A new direction for the speech and language therapy profession. *International Journal of Language & Communication Disorders, 48*(5), 486–496.

Lazarus, R.S. & Folkman, S. (1984). *Stress, Appraisal and Coping*. New York: Springer.

Leahy, M.M. (2004). Therapy talk: Analyzing therapeutic discourse. *Language, Speech, and Hearing Services in Schools, 35*(1), 70–81.

Légaré, F. & Thompson-Leduc, P. (2014). Twelve myths about shared decision making. *Patient Education and Counseling, 96*(3), 281–286. https://doi.org/10.1016/j.pec.2014.06.014

Ley, P. (1988). *Communicating with Patients. Improving Communication, Satisfaction and Compliance*. London: Chapman and Hall.

Ley, P. (1997) (reprint). Communicating with patients: Improving communication, satisfaction, and compliance. Volume 4 of Psychology and Health Series. Maidenhead: Thomas Nelson.

Leventhal, H., Diefenback, M., & Leventhal, E.A. (1992). Illness cognition: Using common sense to understand treatment adherence and affect cognition interactions. *Cognitive Therapy and Research, 16*, 143-163.

Leventhal, H., Safer, M.A., & Panagis, D.M. (1983). The impact of communications on the self-regulations of health beliefs, decisions and behaviour. *Health Education Quarterly, 10*, 3-29.

Liddle, H., James, S., & Hardman, M. (2011). Group therapy for school aged children who stutter: A survey of current practices. *Journal of Fluency Disorders, 36*(4), 274–279.

Lipkin, M., Quill, T., & Napodano, R. (1984). The medical interview: A core curriculum for residencies in internal medicine. *Annals of Internal Medicine, 100*, 277-284.

Lopes, V., Clifford, T., Minnes, P., & Ouellette-Kuntz, H. (2008). Parental stress and coping in families of children with and without developmental delays. *Journal of Developmental Disabilities, 14*, 99-104.

Lott, I., Doran, E., Nguyen, U., Tournay, A., Head, E., & Gillen, D. (2011). Down syndrome and dementia: A randomised controlled trial of antioxidant supplementation. *American Journal of Medical Genetics*, Aug 155A, 1939-1948.

Luborsky, L., Singer, B., & Luborsky, L. (1976). Comparative studies of psychotherapies: Is it true that "everybody has won and all must have prizes"? *Proceedings of the Annual Meeting of the American Psychopathological Association*, 64, 3–22.

Lum, C. (2001). *Scientific Thinking in Speech and Language Therapy, 1st ed*. Mahwah, NJ: Psychology Press.

Lutz, B.J., Young, M.E., Cox, K.J., Martz, C., & Creasy, K.R. (2011). The crisis of stroke: Experiences of patients and their family caregivers. *Topics in Stroke Rehabilitation*, 18(6), 356-368.

Manning, W.H. (2010). Evidence of clinically significant change: The therapeutic alliance and the possibilities of outcomes-informed care. *Seminars in Speech and Language*, 31(4), 207–216.

Manocchi, P. (2017). Fostering academic success in nursing students through mindfulness: A literature review. *Teaching and Learning in Nursing*, 12, 298–303.

Marshall, J. (2000). Critical reflections on the cultural influences in identification and habilitation of children with speech and language difficulties. *International Journal of Disability, Development and Education*, 47(4), 355–369.

Malcomess, K. (2005). The care aims model. In C. Anderson & A. Van der Gaag (Eds). *Speech and Language Therapy: Issues in Professional Practice*. London: Whurr.

Maslach, C. & Jackson, S.E. (1996). *Maslach Burnout Inventory Manual*. Palo Alto, CA: Consulting Psychological Press.

Maslach, C., Scaufell, W.B., & Leiter, M.P. (2001). Job burnout. *Annual Review of Psychology*, 52, 397–422.

Mayer, J.D. & Salovey, P. (1987). What is emotional intelligence? In: P. Salovey & D. Sluyter (Eds), *Emotional Development and Emotional Intelligence: Implications for Educators*. New York: Basic Books.

McConnaughy, E.A., Prochaska, J.O., & Velicer, W.F. (1983). Stages of change in psychotherapy: Measurement and sample profiles. *Psychotherapy: Theory, Research & Practice*, 20(3), 368-375.

McDowell, A. (2014). Health Coaching for Behaviour Change. Interim Progress Report. Health Education East of England. Available from: https://eoeleadership.hee.nhs.uk/sites/default/files/1404813191_LmkH_health_coaching_interim_progress_report.pdf

McDuffie, A., Oakes, A., Machalicek, W., Ma, M., Bullard, L., Nelson, S., & Abbeduto, L. (2016). Early language intervention using distance video-teleconferencing: A pilot study of young boys with Fragile X Syndrome and their mothers. *American Journal of Speech-Language Pathology*, 25(1), 46–66.

McManus, C. (2007). Stress in health professionals. In: S. Ayers, A. Baum, C. McManus, S. Newman, K. Wallston, & J. Weinman (Eds). *Cambridge Handbook of Psychology Health and Medicine*, pp.500-505. Cambridge: Cambridge University Press.

McMullan, M. (2006). Patients using the Internet to obtain health information: How this affects the patient–health professional relationship. *Patient Education and Counseling, 63*(1–2), 24–28.

Mead, N. & Bower, P. (2000). Patient-centredness: A conceptual framework and review of the empirical literature. *Social Science & Medicine, 51*(7), 1087–1110.

Mead, N. & Bower, P. (2002). Patient-centred consultations and outcomes in primary care: A review of the literature. *Patient Education and Counseling, 48*(1), 51–61.

Meleis, A.I. (2011). *Theoretical Nursing: Development and Progress.* New York: Lippincott Williams & Wilkins.

Menzies, R.G., O'Brian, S., Onslow, M., Packman, A., St. Clare, T., & Block, S. (2008). An experimental clinical trial of a cognitive-behavior therapy package for chronic stuttering. *Journal of Speech, Language & Hearing Research, 51*(6), 1451–1464.

Menzies, R.G., Onslow, M., Packman, A., & O'Brian, S. (2009). Cognitive behavior therapy for adults who stutter: A tutorial for speech-language pathologists. *Journal of Fluency Disorders, 34*(3), 187–200.

Merrick, R. & Roulstone, S. (2011). Children's views of communication and speech-language pathology. *International Journal of Speech-Language Pathology, 13*(4), 281–290.

Messer, S. (2004). Evidence-based practice: Beyond empirically supported treatments. *Professional Psychology: Research and Practice, 35,* 580–588.

Michaels, C.E., Michaels, A.J., & Peterson, C. (1997). Motivation and health. In P. Pintrich & M. Maeher (Eds), *Advances in Motivation and Achievement, 10,* 339–374.

Michie, S. & Johnston, M. (2012). Theories and techniques of behaviour change: Developing a cumulative science of behaviour change. *Health Psychology Review, 6*(1), 1–6.

Michie, S., van Stralen, M.M., & West, R. (2011). The Behaviour Change Wheel: A new method for characterising and designing behaviour change interventions. *Implementation Science, 6*(42). https://doi.org/10.1186/1748-5908-6-42

Michie, S., Atkins, L., & West, R. (2014). *The Behaviour Change Wheel: A Guide to Designing Interventions.* Sutton, UK: Silverback Publishing.

Michie, S., Richardson, M., Johnston, M., Abraham, C., Francis, J., Hardeman, W., … Wood, C.E. (2013). The behavior change technique taxonomy (v1) of 93 hierarchically clustered techniques: Building an international consensus for the reporting of behavior change interventions. *Annals of Behavioral Medicine: A Publication of The Society of Behavioral Medicine, 46*(1), 81–95.

Miller, T., Deary, V., & Patterson, J. (2014). Improving access to psychological therapies in voice disorders: A cognitive behavioural therapy model. *Current Opinions in Otolaryngology Head and Neck Surgery, 22*(3), 201–205.

Minnes, P., Perry, A., & Weiss, J.A. (2015). Predictors of distress and well-being in parents of young children with developmental delays and disabilities: The importance of parent perceptions. *Journal of Intellectual Disability Research, 59*(6), 551–560. https://doi.org/10.1111/jir.12160

Mol, A. (2008). *The Logic of Care: Health and the Problem of Patient Choice, 1st ed.* London/ New York: Routledge.

Moos, R.H. & Schaefer, J.A. (1984). The crisis of physical illness: An overview and conceptual approach. In R.H. Moos (Ed.), *Coping with Physical Illness: New Perspectives, 2.* New York: Plenum.

Moran, H. (2012). *Drawing the Ideal Self Manual: A personal construct psychology technique to explore self-esteem.* Retrieved from http://drawingtheidealself.co.uk/drawingtheidealself/ Downloads.html

Morrison, V. & Bennett, P. (2012). *An Introduction to Health Psychology, 3rd ed.* Essex: Pearson Education.

Morrison, T.L. & Smith, J.D. (2013). Working alliance development in occupational therapy: A cross-case analysis. *Australian Occupational Therapy Journal, 60*(5), 326–323. Doi: 10.1111/1440-1630.12053.

Nelson-Jones, R. (2015). *Basic Counselling Skills: A Helper's Manual.* London: Sage.

Naylor, C., Imison, C., Addicott, R., Buck, D., Goodwin, D., Harrison, T., Ross, S., Sonola, L., Tiam, Y., & Curry, N. (2013). *Transforming our Health Care System: Ten Priorities for Commissioners.* London: The King's Fund.

Nazalie, H. & Stringer, H. (2017). Promoting self-reflection and clinical skill development through behaviour change techniques and VEO. Paper presented at National Association of Educators in Practice Conference, Birmingham.

Northcott, S., Burns, K., Simpson, A., & Hilari, K. (2015). Living with aphasia the best I can: A feasibility study exploring solution-focused brief therapy for people with aphasia. *Folia Phoniatrica Logopedica, 67*(3), 156–167.

Nye, C., Vanryckeghem, M., Schwartz, J.B., Herder, C., Turner, H.M., 3rd, & Howard, C. (2013). Behavioral stuttering interventions for children and adolescents: A systematic review and meta-analysis. *Journal of Speech, Language, and Hearing Research, 56*(3), 921–932.

O'Connell, B. (1998). *Solution Focused Therapy.* London: Sage.

O'Connell, B. (2001) *Solution Focused Therapy, 2nd ed.* London: Sage.

Office for National Statistics. (2015). Estimates of the very old (including centenarians): England and Wales and United Kingdon 2002-2014. 30 September 2015. Retrieved from www.statistics.gov.uk

Ogden, J. (2012). *Health Psychology: A Textbook, 5th ed.* Maidenhead: McGraw-Hill Education.

Olkin, R. (1999). *What Therapists Should Know About Disability.* New York: Guilford Press.

Orenstein, E., Basilakos, A., & Marshall, R.S. (2012). Effects of mindfulness meditation on three individuals in aphasia. *International Journal of Language and Communication Disorders, 47*(6), 673–684.

Owens, J. (2015). Creating an impersonal NHS? Personalization, choice and the erosion of intimacy. *Health Expectations, 18*(1), 22–31. https://doi.org/10.1111/hex.12000

Pallesen, H. (2014). Body, coping and self identity. A qualitative 5 year follow up study of stroke. *Disability Rehabilitation, 36*(3), 232–241.

Palmadottir, G. (2006). Client-therapist relationships: Experiences of occupational therapy clients in rehabilitation. *British Journal of Occupational Therapy, 69*(9), 394–401.

Parkinson, K. & Rae, J.P. (1996). The understanding and use of counselling by speech and language therapists at different levels of experience. *European Journal of Disorders of Communication, 31*, 140–152.

Parvizi, J., Archiniegas, D.B., Bernardini, G.L., Hoffman, M.W., et al. (2006). Diagnosis and management of pathological laughter and crying. *Mayo Clinical Proceedings, 81*(11), 1482–1486.

Peterson, C. (2006). *A Primer in Positive Psychology.* Oxford/New York: Oxford University Press, USA.

Peterson, C. & Seligman, M. (2004). *Character Strengths and Virtues. A Handbook and Classification.* Oxford: Oxford University Press.

Petrie, K.J. & Weinman, J. (2006). 2006_why_IPS_matter.pdf. Retrieved April 5, 2017, from https://www.fmhs.auckland.ac.nz/assets/fmhs/som/psychmed/petrie/docs/2006_why_IPS_matter.pdf

Plexico, L.W., Manning, W.H., & DiLollo, A. (2010). Client perceptions of effective and ineffective therapeutic alliances during treatment for stuttering. *Journal of Fluency Disorders, 35*(4), 333–354.

Pomerantz, A.M. (2014). *Clinical Psychology: Science, Practice and Culture, 3rd ed.* Thousand Oaks, CA: Sage Publications.

Por, J. (2005). A pilot data collecting exercise on stress and nursing students. *British Journal of Nursing, 1*, 1180–1184.

Pothier, P., Day, R., Harris, C., & Pothier, D. (2008). Readability statistics of patient information leaflets in a SLT department. *International Journal of Language and Communication Disorders, 43*, 712–722.

Price, P., Kinghorn, J., Patrick, R., & Cardell, B. (2012). "Still there is beauty": One man's resilient adaptation to stroke. *Scandinavian Journal of Occupational Therapy, 19*(2), 111–117.

Prochaska, J.O. & DiClemente, C.C. (1982). Transtheoretical therapy: Toward a more integrative model of change. *Psychotherapy: Theory, Research & Practice, 19*(3), 276–288.

Prochaska, J.O. & DiClemente, C.C. (1986). The transtheoretical approach. In J. Norcross (Ed.), *Handbook of Eclectic Psychotherapy.* New York: Brunner/Mazel.

Prochaska, J.O. & Prochaska, J.M. (1999). Why don't continents move? Why don't people change? *Journal of Psychotherapy Integration, 9*(1), 83–102.

Ratner, N.B. (2006). Evidence-based practice: An examination of its ramifications for the practice of speech-language pathology. *Language, Speech, and Hearing Services in Schools, 37*, 257–267.

Rees, R., Wood, C., & Cavin, K. (2016). Behaviour change techniques, Part 1. *Bulletin*, October 2016, 16–17.

Richardson, A.E., Morton, R., & Broadbent, E. (2015). Caregivers' illness perceptions contribute to quality of life in head and neck cancer patients at diagnosis. *Journal of Psychosocial Oncology, 33*(4), 414–432.

Riley, R. & Weiss, M.C. (2016). A qualitative thematic review: Emotional labour in healthcare settings. *Journal of Advanced Nursing, 72*(1), 6–17.

Robertson, S.A. (2007). Got EQ? Increasing cultural and clinical competence through emotional intelligence. *Communication Disorders Quarterly, 29*(1), 14–19.

Rogers, C. (1951). *Client-Centered Therapy: Its Current Practice, Implications and Theory*. London: Constable.

Rollin, W.J. (1987). *The Psychology of Communication Disorders in Individuals and their Families*. New Jersey: Prentice Hall.

Rosén, A., Lekander, M., Jensen, K., Sachs, L., Petrovic, P., Ingvar, M., & Enblom, A. (2016). The effects of positive or neutral communication during acupuncture for relaxing effects: A sham-controlled randomized trial. *Evidence-Based Complementary & Alternative Medicine (eCAM)*, 1–11.

Rosenzweig, S. (1936). Some implicit common factors in diverse methods of psychotherapy. *American Journal of Orthopsychiatry, 6*, 412–415.

Roulstone, S. & Enderby, P. (2010). The end of an affair: Discharging clients from speech-language pathology. *International Journal of Speech-Language Pathology, 12*(4), 292–295.

Royal College of Speech and Language Therapists. (2009). Curriculum Guidelines. London: RCSLT.

Ruby, M.B., Falk, C.F., Heine, S.J., Villa, C., & Silberstein, O. (2012). Not all collectivisms are equal: Opposing preferences for ideal affect between East Asians and Mexicans. *Emotion, 12*, 1206-1209.

Ruiz-Aranda, D., Extremera, N., & Pineda-Galan, C. (2014). Emotional intelligence, life satisfaction and subjective happiness in female student health professionals: The mediating effects of perceived stress. *Journal of Psychiatric and Mental Health Nursing, 21*, 106-113.

Rvachew, S. & Nowak, M. (2001). The effect of target selection strategy on sound production learning. *Journal of Speech, Language, and Hearing Research, 41*, 172-187.

Sala, F., Krupat, E., & Rother, D. (2002). Satisfaction and the use of humour by physicians and patients. *Psychology and Health, 17*, 269-280.

Santrock, J.W. (2001). *Adolescence, 8th ed*. Boston, MA: McGraw Hill.

Sawbridge, Y. & Hewison, A. (2013). Thinking about the emotional labour of nursing – supporting nurses to care. *Journal of Health Organization and Management, 27*(1), 127–133.

Sandel, M. (2009) Markets and morals. BBC Radio 4. Retrieved from: http://php.york.ac.uk/inst/spru/research/summs/ibsen.php

Schwarzer, R. (1992). Self-efficacy in the adoption and maintenance of health behaviors: Theoretical approaches and a new model. In R. Schwarzer (Ed.), *Self-efficacy: Thought Control of Action* (pp.217–242). Washington, DC: Hemisphere.

Schwarzer, R. & Fuchs, R. (1995). Changing risk behaviors and adopting health behaviors: The role of self-efficacy beliefs. In A. Bandura (Ed.), *Self-efficacy in Changing Societies* (pp.259–288). New York: Cambridge University Press.

Seligman, M. & Csikszentmihalyi, M. (2000). Positive psychology: An introduction. *American Psychologist, 55*(1), 5–14.

Seligman, M.E.P. (2006). *Learned Optimism: How to Change Your Mind and Your Life* (Reprint edition). New York: Vintage Books USA.

Seligman, M.E.P. (2012). *Flourish: A Visionary New Understanding of Happiness and Well-being* (Reprint edition). New York: Atria Books.

Shames, G.H. (2006). *Counselling the Communicatively Disabled and their Families, 2nd ed.* New Jersey: Lawrence Erlbaum.

Sharp, T. (2012). The primacy of positivity: Practical applications for speech-language pathologists. *International Journal of Speech-Language Pathology, 14*(3), 209–213.

Shavitt, S., Cho, Y.I., Johnson, T.P., Jiang, D., Holbrook, A., & Stavrakanonaki, M. (2016). Culture moderates the relation between perceived stress, social support, and mental and physical health. *Journal of Cross-Cultural Psychology, 47*, 956–980.

Shay, L.A. & Lafata, J.E. (2015). Where is the evidence? A systematic review of shared decision making and patient outcomes. *Medical Decision Making: An International Journal of the Society for Medical Decision Making, 35*(1), 114–131. https://doi.org/10.1177/0272989X14551638

Sheeran, P. & Orbell, S. (2000). Using implementation intentions to increase attendance for cervical cancer screening. *Health Psychology, 19*(3), 283–289.

Shrubsole, K., Worrall, L., Power, E., & O'Connor, D. (2016) Recommendations for post stroke aphasia rehabilitation: An updated systematic review and evaluation of clinical practice guidelines. *Aphasiology, 31*(1), 1–124.

Shill, M.A. (1979). Motivational factors in aphasia therapy: Research suggestions. *Journal of Communication Disorders, 12*, 503–517.

Simmons-Mackie, N. & Damico, J.S. (2011). Exploring clinical interaction in speech-language therapy: Narrative, discourse and relationships. In R.J. Fourie (Ed.), *Therapeutic Processes for Communication Disorders: A Guide for Clinicians and Students* (pp.35–52). New York: Psychology Press.

Simpson, S.G. & Reid, C.L. (2014). Therapeutic alliance in videoconferencing psychotherapy: A review. *Australian Journal of Rural Health, 22*(6), 280–299.

Simpson, S., Gale, E., & Denman, A. (2009a). Walking with Dobermans (part 1). *Speech and Language Therapy in Practice*, Autumn 2009, 12–15.

Simpson, S., Gale, E., & Denman, A. (2009b). Walking with Dobermans (part 2). *Speech and Language Therapy in Practice*, Winter 2009, 12–14.

Skolasky, R.L., Mackenzie, E.J., Wegener, S.T., & Riley, L.H., 3rd. (2008). Patient activation and adherence to physical therapy in persons undergoing spine surgery. *Spine, 33*(21), E784–E791.

Smart, J. (2012). *Disability Across the Developmental Lifespan*. New York: Springer.

Sneed, J.R. & Whitbourne, S. (2003). Identity processing and self-consciousness in middle and later adulthood. *The Journal of Gerontology*, *58*(6), 313–319.

Snowden, D. (2002). *Aging with Grace: The Nun Study and the Science of Old Age*. New York: Bantam Books.

Snowling, M., Bishop, D.V.M., Stothard, S.E., Chipchase, B., & Kaplan, C. (2006). Psychosocial outcomes at 15 years of children with a preschool history of speech-language impairment. *Journal of Child Psychology and Psychiatry*, *4*(7), 759–765.

Snyder, C.R. (2002). Hope theory: Rainbows in the mind. *Psychological Inquiry*, 13, 249–275.

Snyder, C.R., Lehman, K.A., Kluck, B., & Monsson, Y. (2006). Hope for rehabilitation and vice versa. *Rehabilitation Psychology*, *51*(2), 89–112.

Solvang, P.K. & Fougner, M. (2016). Professional roles in physiotherapy practice: Educating for self-management, relational matching, and coaching for everyday life. *Physiotherapy Theory and Practice*, *32*(8), 591–602.

Soundy, A., Liles, C., Stubbs, B., & Roskell, C. (2014). Identifying a framework for hope in order to establish the importance of generalised hopes for individuals who have suffered a stroke. *Advances in Medicine*, *2014*, 1–8. https://doi.org/10.1155/2014/471874

Special Education Needs and Disability Act (2001). http://www.legislation.gov.uk

Stewart, M. (2002). Cultural competence in undergraduate healthcare education: Review of the issues. *Physiotherapy*, *88*(10), 620–629.

Stewart, M., Brown, J., Weston, W., McWhinney, I., McWilliam, C., & Freeman, T. (1995). *Patient-centred Medicine: Transforming the Clinical Method*. London: Sage.

Stringer, H. & Toft, K. (2016a). Behaviour change techniques part 1. *Bulletin*, November 2016, 24–25.

Stringer, H. & Toft, K. (2016b). Behaviour change techniques part 2. *Bulletin*, December 2016, 18–19.

Stroebe, M. & Schutt, H. (1999). The dual process model of coping with bereavement: rationale and description. *Death Studies*, *23*, 197–224.

Svetaz, M.V., Ireland, M., & Blum, R. (2001). Adolescents with learning disabilities: Risk and protective factors associated with emotional well-being. Findings from the National Longitudinal Study of Adolescent Health. *Journal of Adolescent Health*, *28*(4), 355.

Syder, D. & Levy, C. (1998). Personal supervision. In: D. Syder (Ed.), *Wanting to Talk*. London: Whurr.

www.talkmebetter.co.uk

Taylor, R.R. (2008). *The Intentional Relationship. Occupational Therapy and the Use of Self*. Philadelphia: FA Davis.

Tan, S. S.-L. & Goonawardene, N. (2017). Internet health information seeking and the patient-physician relationship: A systematic review. *Journal of Medical Internet Research*, *19*(1), 1-15.

Tervalon, M. & Murray-Garcia, J. (1998). Cultural humility versus cultural competence: A critical distinction in defining physician training outcomes in multicultural education. *Journal of Healthcare for the Poor and the Undeserved, 9*, 117-125.

Thomas, S., Walker, M.F., Macniven, J.A., Haworth, H., & Lincoln, N. (2013). Communication and low mood (CALM): A randomised controlled trial of behavioural therapy for stroke patients with aphasia. *Clinical Rehabilitation, 27* (5), 398-408.

Thyme, K. & Frøkjær-Jensen, B. (2001). *The Accent Method: A Rational Voice Therapy in Theory & Practice*. Milton Keynes: Speechmark.

Timmins, F., Corroon, A.M., Byrne, G., & Mooney, B. (2011). The challenge of contemporary nurse education programmes. Perceived stressors of nursing students: Mental health and related lifestyle issues. *Journal of Psychiatric and Mental Health Nursing, 18*(9), 758-766.

Togher, L. (2010). The dilemma of discharge and some possible solutions. *International Journal of Speech-Language Pathology, 12*(4), 320-324.

Turkstra, L.S. (2000). Should my shirt be tucked in or left out? The communication context of adolescence. *Aphasiology, 14*(4), 349-364.

Turkstra, L.S., Williams, W.H., Tonks, J., & Frampton, I. (2008). Measuring social cognition in adolescents: Implications for students with TBI returning to school. *Neurorehabilitation, 23*(6), 501-509.

Turnbull, J. (2000). The transtheoretical model of change: Examples from stammering. *Counselling Psychology Quarterly, 31*(1), 13-21.

Twiddy, M., House, A., & Jones, F. (2012). The association between discrepancy in illness representations on distress in stroke patients and carers. *Journal of Psychosomatic Research, 72*(3), 220-225.

van Leer, E. & Connor, N.P. (2015). Predicting and influencing voice therapy adherence using social-cognitive factors and mobile video. *American Journal of Speech-Language Pathology, 24*(2), 164-176.

van Wilgen, P., Beetsma, A., Neels, H., Roussel, N., & Nijs, J. (2014). Physical therapists should integrate illness perceptions in their assessment in patients with chronic musculoskeletal pain: A qualitative analysis. *Manual Therapy, 19*(3), 229-234.

Verdon, S., Wong, S., & McLeod, S. (2016). Shared knowledge and mutual respect: Enhancing culturally competent practice through collaboration with families and communities. *Child Language Teaching and Therapy, 32*(2), 205-221.

Villeneuve, M., Chatenoud, C., Hutchinson, N., Minnes, P., Perry A., Dionne, C. et al. (2013). The experience of parents as their children with developmental disabilities transition from early intervention to kindergarten. *Canadian Journal of Education, 36*, 14-43.

Vinney, L.A. & Turkstra, L.S. (2013). The role of self-regulation in voice therapy. *Journal of Voice, 27*(3), 390.

Vinney, L.A., van Mersbergen, M., Connor, N.P., & Turkstra, L.S. (2016). Vocal control: Is it susceptible to the negative effects of self-regulatory depletion? *Journal of Voice, 30*(5), 638.

Vohs, K.D. & Baumeister, R.F. (2004). Depletion of self-regulatory resources makes people selfish. Unpublished manuscript, University of British Columbia, Vancouver, BC, Canada.

Wampold, B.E. (2001). *The Great Psychotherapy Debate: Models, Methods, and Findings.* Mahwah, NJ: Lawrence Erlbaum.

Wampold, B.E. (2015). How important are the common factors in psychotherapy? An update. *World Psychiatry, 14*(3), 270–277.

Wampold, B.E., Minami, T., Baskin, T.W., & Callen Tierney, S. (2002). A meta-(re)analysis of the effects of cognitive therapy versus "other therapies" for depression. *Journal of Affective Disorders, 68*(2–3), 159–165.

Ward, E.C., Sharma, S., Burns, C., Theodoros, D., Russell, T., Ward, E.C., & Russell, T. (2012). Validity of conducting clinical dysphagia assessments for patients with normal to mild cognitive impairment via telerehabilitation. *Dysphagia, 27*(4), 460–472.

Ward, R.A. (2010). How old am I? Perceived age in middle and later life. *International Journal of Ageing and Human Development, 71*(3), 167-184.

Watts Pappas, N., McAllister, L., & McLeod, S. (2016). Parental beliefs and experiences regarding involvement in intervention for their child with speech sound disorder. *Child Language Teaching and Therapy, 32*(2), 223–239.

Weaver, A.D. & Allen, J.A. (2017). Emotional labor and the work of school psychologists. *Contemporary School Psychology*, 1–11.

White, J.H., Magin, P., Attia, J., Sturm, J., Carter, G., & Pollack, M. (2012). Trajectories of psychological distress after stroke. *Annals of Family Medicine, 10*(5), 435–442.

Whitbourne, S.K. (1986). *The Me I Know: A Study of Adult Identity.* New York: Springer-Verlag.

Whitehouse, A.J.O., Hird, K., & Cocks, N. (2007). The recruitment and retention of speech and language therapists: What do university students find important? *Journal of Allied Health, 36*(3), 131–136.

Wilkinson, R. (2004). Reflecting on talk in speech and language therapy: Some contributions using conversation analysis. *International Journal of Language & Communication Disorders, 39*(4), 497–503.

Williams, A. (2013). The strategies used to deal with emotion work in student paramedic practice. *Nurse Education in Practice, 13*(3), 207–212. https://doi.org/10.1016/j.nepr.2012.09.010

Williams, S. & Murray, C. (2013). The lived experience of older adults' occupational adaptation following a stroke. *Australian Occupational Therapy Journal, 60*(1), 39–47.

Wilson, P. (1988). *Games without Frontiers.* London: Marshall Pickering.

Wilson, P. & Long, I. (2009). *The Big Book of Blob Trees.* Abington-on-Thames: Routledge.

Wittig, A.F. & Schurr, K.T. (1994). Psychological characteristics of women volleyball players: Relationships with injuries, rehabilitation, and team success. *Personality and Social Psychology Bulletin, 20*, 322–323.

Wolever, R.Q., Simmons, L.A., Sforzo, G.A., Dill, D., Kaye, M., Bechard, E.M., … Yang, N. (2013). A systematic review of the literature on health and wellness coaching: Defining a key behavioral intervention in healthcare. *Global Advances in Health and Medicine, 2*(4), 38–57. https://doi.org/10.7453/gahmj.2013.042

Wolter, J.A., DiLollo, A., & Apel, K. (2006). A narrative therapy approach to counselling: A model for working with adolescents and adults with language-literacy deficits. *Language, Speech, and Hearing Services in the Schools, 37,*168-177.

Woodrow, P. (2002). *Ageing: Issues for Physical, Psychological and Social Health.* London: Whurr.

World Health Organisation. (2015). Healthy ageing. http://www.who.int/ageing/events/world-report-2015-launch/en/

World Health Organisation. (2015). Adolescents: Health risks and solutions. Factsheet N°345. Updated May 2014.

Yalom, I.D. & Leszcz, M. (2005). *The Theory and Practice of Group Psychotherapy.* New York: Basic Books.

Ylvisaker, M. & Feeney. T. (2000). Reflections on Dobermanns, poodles, and social rehabilitation for difficult to serve individuals with traumatic brain injury. *Aphasiology, 14*(4), 407-431.

Ylvisaker, M. & Feeney, T. (2002). Executive functions, self-regulation, and learned optimism in paediatric rehabilitation: A review and implications for intervention. *Pediatric Rehabilitation, 5*(2), 51-70.

Ylvisaker, M., McPherson, K., Kayes, N., & Pellett, E. (2008). Metaphoric identity mapping: Facilitating goal setting and engagement in rehabilitation after traumatic brain injury. *Neuropsychological Rehabilitation, 18*(5-6), 713-741.

Young Dementia UK. https://www.youngdementiauk.org/

Zebrowski, P.M. & Arenas, R.M. (2011). The "Iowa Way" revisited. *Journal of Fluency Disorders, 36*(3), 144-157.

Index